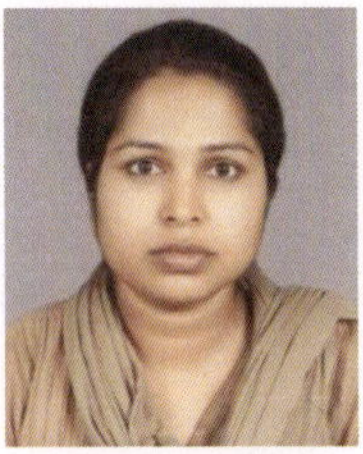

Dr. Neelam Kushwaha is presently working as an Associate Professor (Veterinary Medicine) at College of Veterinary and Animal Sciences, Bihar Animal Sciences University, Kishanganj. Earlier, she served at College of Veterinary and Animal Sciences, Maharashtra Animal and Fishery Sciences University, Udgir, as Hospital Registrar (Veterinary Clinical Medicine, Ethics, and Jurisprudence) over a period of seven years. She did her BVSc&AH and MVSc from GBPUA&T, Pantnagar. She was awarded PhD in Veterinary Medicine from ICAR-IVRI, Izatnagar.

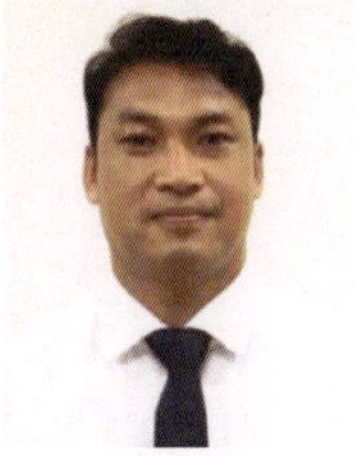

Dr. Raju Kumar Dewry is presently working as Assistant Professor (Veterinary Gynaecology and Obstetrics) at College of Veterinary and Animal Sciences, Bihar Animal Sciences University, Kishanganj, since March 30, 2023. He did his BVSc&AH and MVSc (Animal Reproduction, Gynaecology and Obstetrics) from College of Veterinary Science, Assam Agricultural University, and PhD in Veterinary Gynaecology and Obstetrics from ICAR-National Dairy Research Institute, Karnal. His area of interest is andrology. He had published 20 research papers in various journals and received four awards.

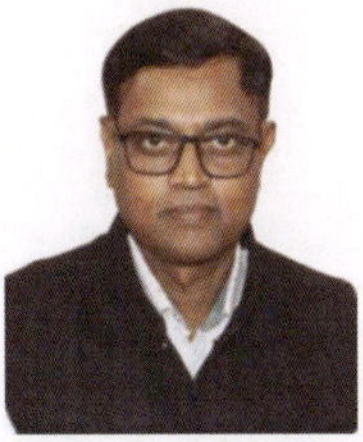

Dr. Chandrahas, is presently working as Dean, College of Veterinary and Animal Sciences (CoVAS), Kishanganj, since 24.11.2022. He has more than 22 years' experience of Teaching, Research, Innovation and Extension. He has authored more than 350 publications including 64 research articles, 15 books, 20 practical manuals, 37 book chapters, 52 popular articles, 05 Technical Bulletin, 30 lead papers, 55 research abstracts, 53 MOUs etc. Registration of 04 native chicken varities and 03 patents are in pipeline. He has received 34 awards including Gold Medals, JRF, SRF, ARS, Young Scientist, Best paper, Best poster awards etc. He has been awarded Fellow National of Animal Production and Management (FNAPM) by ISAPM in 2019. He has guided 04 M.V.Sc. and 06 Ph.D. students as major advisor. He has handled 19 research projects including PI in 09 projects. His one of the notable area of work is management of Poultry and Piggery Wastes. He has developed 'DAC' Technology for all-weather bio-gas production exclusively from both layer and broiler type of poultry excreta.

Veterinary First Aid

Vineet Kumar
Associate Professor
Department of Veterinary Surgery and Radiology
College of Veterinary and Animal Sciences
Bihar Animal Sciences University
Kishanganj-855107, Bihar, India

Anand Mohan
Assistant Professor (Veterinary Medicine)
Department of Veterinary Veterinary Clinical Complex
College of Veterinary and Animal Sciences
Bihar Animal Sciences University
Kishanganj-855107, Bihar, India

Neelam Kushwaha
Associate Professor
Department of Veterinary Medicine
College of Veterinary and Animal Sciences
Bihar Animal Sciences University
Kishanganj-855107, Bihar, India

Raju Kumar Dewry
Assistant Professor
Department of Veterinary Gynaecology and Obstetrics
Bihar Animal Sciences University
Kishanganj-855107, Bihar, India

Chandrahas
Dean
College of Veterinary and Animal Sciences
Bihar Animal Sciences University
Kishanganj-855107, Bihar, India

NIPA® GENX ELECTRONIC RESOURCES & SOLUTIONS P. LTD.
New Delhi-110 034

NIPA® GENX ELECTRONIC
RESOURCES & SOLUTIONS P. LTD.

101,103, Vikas Surya Plaza, CU Block
L.S.C.Market, Pitam Pura, New Delhi-110 034
Ph : +91 11 27341616, 27341717, 27341718
E-mail: newindiapublishingagency@gmail.com
www: www.nipabooks.com

For customer assistance, please contact
Phone: + 91-11-27 34 17 17
Fax: + 91-11-27 34 16 16

Print ISBN: 978-93-58878-23-3

ebook ISBN: 978-93-58877-16-8

Composed and Designed by NIPA®.

बिहार पशु विज्ञान विश्वविद्यालय
बिहार पशु चिकित्सा महाविद्यालय प्रांगण, पटना - 800014
BIHAR ANIMAL SCIENCES UNIVERSITY
BIHAR VETERINARY COLLEGE CAMPUS, PATNA – 800014

डॉ० रामेशवर सिंह
कुलपति
Dr. Rameshwar Singh
Vice-Chancellor

☎ : 0612-2222221
: +91-94728-64654
E-mail : vc-basu-bih@gov.in
vicechancellorbasu@gmail.com

FOREWORD

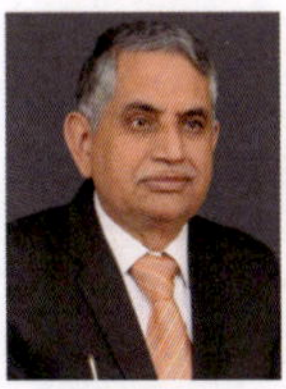

It is with great pleasure and admiration that I introduce the "Veterinary First Aid," a comprehensive field reference guide meticulously crafted by thirteen distinguished faculty members from the College of Veterinary and Animal Sciences, Bihar Animal Sciences University, Kishanganj. This handbook stands as a testament to their unwavering commitment to advancing veterinary science and providing practical, life-saving knowledge to veterinarians, animal health workers, and animal caretakers in the field.

Veterinary first aid is an essential skill set, bridging the gap between the onset of an injury or illness and the arrival of professional medical care. The need for immediate and effective first aid interventions cannot be overstated, especially in rural and remote areas where access to veterinary hospitals may be limited. This handbook serves as an indispensable resource, offering clear, concise, and actionable information on a wide range of emergency situations that veterinarians and animal caregivers may encounter.

In addition to its practical applications, the "Veterinary First Aid" reflects the broader mission of Bihar Animal Sciences University to promote animal welfare and enhance the quality of veterinary education and practice. By equipping animal health professionals with the knowledge and skills to perform first aid effectively, this handbook contributes to the overall improvement of animal health and well-being in the community.

I commend the authors for their dedication and hard work in producing this valuable resource, and I am confident that it will have a profound and lasting impact on the field of veterinary medicine.

21.5.24

(Rameshwar Singh)

Preface

This edition of the **Veterinary First Aid** is written with a broad view to provide concise but valuable and necessary information for animal owners, practicing veterinarians, and paraveterinarians. This book has been written by thirteen faculties from the College of Veterinary and Animal Sciences, Bihar Animal Sciences University, Kishanganj, after receiving feedback from animal owners during Kissan Samvad and animal health camps. This book contains 37 chapters covering commonly encountered clinical conditions at the field level and their first aid. Each chapter generally covers an overview of key points, an introduction, etiologies, clinical findings, possible first aid given at the animal site, and suggested references.

Every effort was made by the contributors to incorporate their real-time practical experience into this book in addition to their theoretical knowledge to make effective communication that will be useful to the readers.

Editors

Contents

III Poisoning

IV Miscellaneous

List of Contributors

1. **Abhishek Kumar, MVSc, PhD**
   Assistant Professor, Veterinary Gyanecology and Obstetrics
   College of Veterinary and Animal Sciences
   Bihar Animal Sciences University
   Kishanganj-855107 (Bihar)

2. **Anand Mohan, MVSc, PhD**
   Assistant Professor, Veterinary Medicine
   College of Veterinary and Animal Sciences
   Bihar Animal Sciences University
   Kishanganj-855107 (Bihar)

3. **Diptimayee Sahoo, MVSc, PhD**
   Assistant Professor, Veterinary Pathology
   College of Veterinary and Animal Sciences
   Bihar Animal Sciences University
   Kishanganj-855107 (Bihar)

4. **Komal, MVSc**
   Assistant Professor, Veterinary Biochemistry
   College of Veterinary and Animal Sciences
   Bihar Animal Sciences University
   Kishanganj-855107 (Bihar)

5. **Kumari Chandrakala, MVSc**
   Assistant Professor, Veterinary Surgery and Radiology
   College of Veterinary and Animal Sciences
   Bihar Animal Sciences University
   Kishanganj-855107 (Bihar)

6. **Mamta Mishra, MVSc, PhD**
   Assistant Professor, Veterinary Surgery and Radiology
   College of Veterinary and Animal Sciences
   Bihar Animal Sciences University
   Kishanganj-855107 (Bihar)

7. **Nancy Jasrotia, MVSc**
   Assistant Professor, Veterinary Gyanecology and Obstetrics
   College of Veterinary and Animal Sciences
   Bihar Animal Sciences University
   Kishanganj-855107 (Bihar)

8. **Neelam Kushwaha, MVSc, PhD**
Associate Professor, Veterinary Medicine
College of Veterinary and Animal Sciences
Bihar Animal Sciences University
Kishanganj-855107 (Bihar)

9. **Pratyush Kumar, MVSc**
Assistant Professor, Veterinary Gyanecology and Obstetrics
College of Veterinary and Animal Sciences
Bihar Animal Sciences University
Kishanganj-855107 (Bihar)

10. **Raju Kumar Dewry, MVSc, PhD**
Assistant Professor, Veterinary Gyanecology and Obstetrics
College of Veterinary and Animal Sciences
Bihar Animal Sciences University
Kishanganj-855107 (Bihar)

11. **Richa Arora, MVSc, PhD**
Assistant Professor, Veterinary Biochemistry
College of Veterinary and Animal Sciences
Bihar Animal Sciences University
Kishanganj-855107 (Bihar)

12. **Safeeda Sultana Begum, MVSc, PhD**
Assistant Professor, Veterinary Medicine
College of Veterinary and Animal Sciences
Bihar Animal Sciences University
Kishanganj-855107 (Bihar)

13. **S. Ramanarayanan, MVSc, PhD**
Assistant Professor, Veterinary Pharmacology and Toxicology
College of Veterinary and Animal Sciences
Bihar Animal Sciences University
Kishanganj-855107 (Bihar)

I General

1

Assessment of Patients

Anand Mohan

Key Points

- Patient assessment is only half of the disease diagnosis process.
- Using animal physiological values as a reference point can help measure a patient's health.
- Laboratory results support the patient's evaluation results.
- Patient evaluation findings suggest bodily system involvement.

Introduction

The patient assessment includes the owner's complaint, history, physical examination, and clinical examination of the animals (Fig. 1.1). Proper animal assessment is only part of the illness diagnosis process. Sometimes, evaluation results can be indicative of a medical condition. As a result, at the initial stage, assessing the animal aids in making a confirmation diagnosis. Given its significance, an assessment of the animal must be performed or obtained before concluding the laboratory finding, if available. Assessment can be conducted in several steps, each of which is detailed in the next paragraph. The physiological vital parameters of animals are crucial reference points to conclude the evaluation findings.

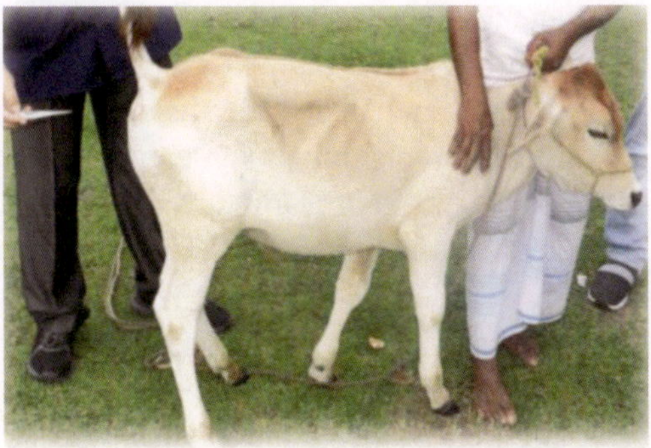

Fig. 1.1. Image showing clinical examination of a Purnea cattle calf.

Table 1.1. Normal physiological values of vital parameters

Sr. No.	Species	Temperature (°F)	Pulse /min	Respiration / min	Ruminal movement / 5 min
1.	Cow & Buffaloes	101.0 – 102.0	40 - 60	12 - 16	5 - 8
2.	Horses	100.0 – 101.0	30 - 40	8 - 12	-
3.	Sheep & Goats	103.0 – 104.0	55 - 75	20 - 30	6 - 9
4.	Pig	102.0 – 103.0	60 - 75	20 - 30	6 - 9
5.	Dog	101.0 – 102.0	80 - 100	15 - 25	-
6.	Cats	101.0 – 102.0	110 - 120	20 - 40	-
7.	Fowl	106.0 -107.0	120 - 160	15 - 50	-

(*Source*: Textbook of Clinical Veterinary Medicine by MC Sharma, Mahesh Kumar, and RD Sharma, Directorate of Information and Publications of Agriculture, ICAR., January 2009, Appendix I, PP 604).

Physical examination

Routine physical examinations of animals include taking a history, inspecting the environment, and inspecting the patient. Inadequate evaluation of any of these can result in errors in diagnosis.

1. ***History-taking*** is the most important component of a physical examination. It aids in the precise diagnosis of diseases and provides a proper prognosis. It includes: a) patient information; b) disease history; and c) general history.

Patient data includes information about the species, breed, sex, and age of the animal. The susceptibility of animals to disease varies significantly depending on species, age, breed, and sex. As a result, information from patient data provides insights for diagnosis. Cattle and buffalo, for example, are susceptible to hemorrhagic septicemia (HS), black quarter (BQ), rinderpest (RP), bovine viral diarrohea (BVD), bovine malignant catarrhal (BMC) fever, ephemeral fever, traumatic reticuloperitonitis (TRP), traumatic pericarditis, diaphragmatic hernia (DH), and so on. Sheep and goats are susceptible to peste des petits ruminants (PPR), contagious ecthyma, blue tongue, pregnancy toxemia, fibrinous pericarditis, enterotoxemia, and so on. Dogs are susceptible to rabies, canine distemper (CD), infectious canine hepatitis (ICH), diabetes, chronic valvular disease, and so on. Pigs are susceptible to swine fever, swine erysipelas, and swine influenza. Horses are susceptible to glander, strangle, equine infectious anemia (EIA), African horse sickness (AHS), equine influenza, and so on. Similarly, the sex and breed of animals might influence the development of some diseases.

Mastitis, metritis, pyometra, milk fever, ketosis, and pregnancy toxemia are common in female animals, whereas male animals can develop orchitis, scrotal hernia, phimosis, paraphimosis, urolithiasis, and horn cancer. Exotic breeds are more prone to foot-and-mouth disease (FMD) and hemoprotozoal illness, for example. Jerseys are more susceptible to milk fever. High-yielding animals are prone to metabolic and production diseases. Age is another variable in patient data. Some diseases are more common in young animals, such as colibacilosis, naval ill, coccidiosis, ascariasis, dermatophytosis, rickets, tetanus, and so on (cattle and buffalo), enterotoxemia, lamb dysentery, tetanus, endoparasites, and so on (sheep and goat), strangles (horse), piglet anemia (pig), canine distemper, rickets, and ringworm (dogs). Similarly, diseases that affect old animals include tuberculosis, Johne's disease (JD), osteomalacia, TRP, DH (cattle and buffalo), diabetes mellitus, prostitis (dogs), and glanders.

Disease history contains both current/immediate disease and past/previous disease-related information. In the case of the current medical condition, an attempt should be made to obtain information on the clinical abnormalities noted by the owner in the order in which they arose. A faulty disease history may lead to clinical errors. The clinician should arrange the chronological order of clinical indications revealed by the owner through patient assessment and subject expertise.

Examples include the duration of illness, changes in hunger, water intake, defecation, urination, rumination, respiration, and growth in young animals, as well as milk production in lactating animals, physical activity, stride, and posture. Morbidity, case fatality, and population mortality rate, past exposure, prior treatment, prophylactic and control methods used, and transit time should be considered. If there is a history of previous illness or diseases, inquire about the nature and duration of the previous illness, morbidity, mortality, and case fatality rates, clinical signs observed, laboratory tests performed, diagnosis made, proper treatment given, control measures implemented such as vaccination, deworming, and spraying, and results obtained.

General history includes (a) nutrition: the quality and quantity of feed and water given to the animal aid in diagnosis. For example, overfeeding green or lush pasture causes tympany or diarrhea, but feeding low-quality fodder causes rumen impaction; (b) breeding: A history of parturition or pregnancy implies or rules out diagnostic options. Pregnancy toxemia occurs in advanced pregnant sheep; metritis occurs within a few days after parturition; and milk fever commonly occurs within 48-72 hours of parturition in cows and buffaloes; and (c) housing/climate: information on the season of occurrence, topography, environmental temperature, humidity, rainfall, and so on aids in the diagnosis of specific diseases, such as heat stroke, which occurs in animals exposed to extremely high temperatures. Surra, blue tongue, and ephemeral fever are vector-borne diseases that are associated with excessive rainfall.

Examination of the environment

Outdoor factors such as topography and soil type, stocking rate (population density), waste disposal, and feed and water supply should be evaluated, while hygiene, ventilation, flooring, lighting, and so on should be examined in the inside environment. High population density is a predisposing cause of disease because the buildup of urine and feces increases the risk of infection.

2. ***Examination of patient*:** Each patient should get a general clinical evaluation. Each animal should be thoroughly examined. Excluding examination of any area of the body leads to an incorrect diagnosis. Physical examinations consist of four components. It entails observation, palpation, percussion, and auscultation. A thorough assessment of many body systems, as well as laboratory tests, is necessary.
    a. *Inspection (distant examination):* Inspection is a visual check of the animal from a distance that does not upset the patient. Many observations, such as changes in behavior and appearance, should be carefully recorded. The examination includes an assessment of behavior, excitation states, voice, feed intake, defecation, urination, posture, gait, body condition, body conformation, skin, and other factors.
    b. *Palpation:* It is the physical handling of an animal's tissues, organs, or body components. The tip or ball of the finger is most commonly employed in palpation to identify the form, size, position, and structure of an organ; the existence and degree of pain; the consistency of a lesion; the temperature and sensitivity of a lesion or organ, and so on. Small and medium-sized animals are most suited for internal organ palpation. Cattle, buffalo, and horses have big bodies, making it difficult to palpate their internal organs. Palpation is best performed with the animal standing, but it can also be done in a reclined position, especially with dogs and cats. First, palpate the neighboring healthy area of the lesion, then the lesion itself.

Palpation is not particularly useful in detecting thoracic organ problems. Use a flat hand to feel the heartbeat on the left side of the chest, between the fourth and sixth intercostal gaps. Abnormalities can be diagnosed by palpating the rumen on the left flank. Small animals' internal organs can be palpated. On the right side of the abdomen, the liver can be felt. Digital pressure can be used to feel the intestines in cats and dogs. Superficial lymph nodes, such as pre-scapular, pre-femoral, and supra-mammary lymph nodes, are easily palpable. Retropharyngeal, submandibular, and parotid lymph nodes can only be palpated when they are swollen. Rectal palpation in large animals such as cows, buffaloes, and horses can reveal information on the digestive, reproductive, and urinary tracts. The goal of the rectal palpation or examination is to detect any abdominal organ abnormalities that are not obvious during a routine clinical examination. It should be done carefully to avoid harm by using an appropriate lubricant.

Types of palpation

a) ***Direct palpation:*** It is done with finger tips or the palm.

b) ***Indirect palpation:*** It is done with a probe, catheter, or any such instrument. It is used when a body part is out of the hand's reach.

   On the basis of palpation, the consistency of tissue, organ, or swelling can be classified as follows:

   - *Doughy* - this occurs when the structure pits under pressure, as in edema.
   - *Firm* – when the structure resembles that of a normal liver.
   - *Hard* – when structures have a bone-like consistency.
   - *Fluctuating* - structures are soft, elastic, and undulate with pressure but do not retain finger imprints.
   - *Tension* - occurs when the structure feels like a viscus filled with gas or fluid under high pressure.
   - *Emphysema* - is characterized by puffy and bloated structures that crackle under pressure due to gas in the tissue.

c) ***Percussion:*** Striking the body surface causes deep portions to vibrate and produce audible sounds. An audible resonance provides essential information regarding the position, size, and consistency of the structure impacted. It helps to diagnose diseases in the lungs, rumen, and other abdominal organs. However, it has minimal application for fatty animals such as buffaloes. It may not be useful for determining the health state of deeply seated organs.

Percussion can be completed in two different ways: (a) Horizontal percussion stage- This is performed from the anterior to the posterior of the lung. This helps to distinguish the lung region from the adjacent hepatic and omasal dullness on the right side and rumen resonance on the left in cattle, and (b) Vertical percussion stage- This is carried out at each intercostal space, beginning at the top border of the lung and progressing downward. Identifying the region of dullness, relative cardiac dullness, and emphysema is beneficial.

Types of percussion

a) **Direct or immediate percussion:** involves striking a body part directly with the fingertips or a plexor or hammer.

b) **Indirect or mediate percussion involves:** placing the left hand's fingers flat on a part of the body and striking it with the right hand's flexed middle finger or a pleximeter and hammer.

Percussion sounds: the sound produced by percussion can be defined as:

a) *Resonant* - the sound generated by air-filled organs, such as the normal lung.

b) *Tympanitic* - A drum-like tone generated by an organ carrying gas under pressure, such as the rumen or cecum.

c) *Dull* - the sound made by solid organs like the heart and liver.

Modified percussions

a) ***Ballotment:*** Detects floating viscera or masses in the abdominal cavity. Using extended fingers or a clenched fist, the abdominal wall is vigorously palpated with a hard push to drive the organ or mass away and then allowed to rebound onto the fingertips. It assists in the diagnosis of carbohydrate engorgement and excessive amounts of fluid in the rumen, or left-side displacement of the abomasum, intestinal obstruction, abomasal volvulus, cecal dilatation and torsion, and paralytic ileus.

b) ***Tactile percussion:*** A combination of percussion and palpation. It consists of percussion on one side of the abdominal wall and palpation on the other side of the belly to detect fluid waves. It helps to determine the fluid in the peritoneal cavity, e.g., ascites and uroperitoneum.

Auscultation

Auscultation is the process of listening for normal noises produced by organ movement such as the lung, gut, and heart. Auscultation is beneficial for examining the lung, pleura, trachea, heart, and several areas of the digestive system. It aids in the detection of disorders of the lungs and heart, such as pneumonia, pleurisy, pericarditis, and endocarditis. Auscultation can be used to assess a gravid uterus. Direct auscultation is accomplished by placing the ear on the body's surface over the organ. Direct auscultation is harmful in ferocious animals and is not recommended for health reasons. Indirect auscultation is accomplished with a stethoscope, phonendoscope, or electronic stethoscope. This technique is more effective than direct auscultation.

The heart is positioned in the ventral thorax, between the third and sixth ribs on the left side. The rate, rhythm, and cardiac sounds must be carefully interpreted. The lung auscultation area is a triangle formed by the caudal angle of the scapula, the olecranon process of the ulna, and the second last intercostal space at the point of a horizontal line drawn from the external angle of the scapula to the external angle of the ileum, i.e., tuber coxae (16th rib in horses and 11th in cattle, buffalo, sheep, goat, and dog). Rumen contractions can be heard by placing a stethoscope on the left paralumbar fossa. Normal rumen contractions (1-3 per minute) are powerful and easily felt.

References

A text book of the diseases of cattle, sheep, pigs, goats and horses by Rodostis O. M., Gay C. C., Blood D. C. and Hinchcliff K.W., 9th edition, Saunders Publication.

Textbook of Clinical Veterinary Medicine by MC Sharma, Mahesh Kumar and RD Sharma, Directorate of Information and Publications of Agriculture, ICAR., January 2009.

II Emergencies

2

Allergic Reactions

Safeeda Sultana Begum

Key Points

- Allergies are widespread among animals.
- Common allergens include food and drugs.
- Allergic reactions can occur through inhalation, skin contact, or eating.
- Housed cattle develop hypersensitivity pneumonitis, a persistent respiratory illness.
- Chronic exposure to spores in moldy, dusty hay is linked to the disease.
- There are two types of hypersensitivity: acute (also known as anaphylaxis or shock) and delayed.

Introduction

Anaphylaxis is a severe, immediate-type reaction that affects the cutaneous, respiratory, cardiovascular, and gastrointestinal systems within minutes to an hour after contact with a precipitating substance. Lethal anaphylaxis is characterized by severe (upper or lower) airway blockage, shock, and extreme hypotension.

Etiology

Severe anaphylactic reactions are prevalent in farm animals following the injection of drugs or biological products such as sera and bacterins. recurrent intravenous injection of specific items, medications, or vaccinations (usually following the administration of conventional drugs or test agents); or recurrent blood transfusion from the same donor. Ingestion of some pasture feeds or fodders, as well as certain allergen-containing foods, can trigger anaphylaxis, which can be fatal if not treated promptly. Sometimes, drying animals or bagged-up animals (for exhibition) demonstrate milk allergy, and in specific species, an allergic reaction may develop due to the death of *Hypoderma* spp. larvae in the animal's cutaneous tissue.

Clinical findings

The earliest symptoms of an anaphylactic reaction include sudden and acute dyspnea, muscular shaking, and anxiety. Severe muscle tremors may cause a fever to rise. In cases of pulmonary oedema, auscultation may indicate an increased vesicular murmur and crackling sounds. Other clinical indications, such as copious salivation, mild bloating, and diarrhea, are reported in some cases of anaphylactic reactions.

Treatment

The treatment of allergic conditions, particularly anaphylaxis, is predicated on the rapid treatment of inflammation or allergy symptoms, which is usually accomplished by administering epinephrine, corticosteroids, and antihistamines and avoiding further exposure to the inciting allergen. Epinephrine injected intramuscularly is frequently instantly effective. However, most anaphylactic reactions are of moderate severity and resolve spontaneously in otherwise healthy animals within minutes or a few hours. Corticosteroids should be administered soon after epinephrine to preserve vascular integrity and reduce pulmonary vessel permeability. Acetylsalicylic acid was found to be more effective than antihistamines in treating experimental anaphylaxis in cattle and horses.

If there are signs of probable pulmonary edema, oxygen should be administered as soon as possible, ideally under positive pressure, to avoid airway blockage. In the event of inflammation, NSAIDs such as flunixin meglumine, phenylbutazone, and meclofenamic acid can be used.

References

https://www.msdvetmanual.com/respiratory-system/non-infectious-respiratory-system-diseases-in-cattle/hypersensitivity-pneumonitis-in-cattle

Radostits, O. M., Gay, C. C., Blood, D. C. and Hinchcliff, K. W. (2000). Veterinary Medicine: A textbook of cattle, sheep, pigs, goats and horses, nona edizione. Saunders, London, UK.

3

Animal Bites and Stings

Neelam Kushwaha

Key Points

- Animal bites containing poisons, venoms, or diseases cause significant morbidity and mortality.
- Unattended animals are vulnerable to various types of bites, including snakes, spiders, scorpions, bee stings, lizards, and dogs.
- Snake bites can be life-threatening for both humans and animals and require emergency treatment.
- Dog bites can cause rabies in both people and animals.

Introduction

If left alone, curious animals are likely to be bitten by a variety of insects. Bite severity varies by animal species. Typically, stings and bites are painful and dangerous. It can be life-threatening in certain situations.

Snake Bite

- Spider bite
- Scorpions bite
- Bees sting
- Lizard bite
- Dog bite

Snake Bite

Snake bites are well-known veterinary emergencies. Cattle, buffalo, sheep, goats, and horses graze in fields and pastures, disrupting snakes and other pests as they go through their habitats. It is also prevalent in dogs. Snake bites are rare in pigs because of their thick fat layer. Large animals (such as cattle, buffaloes, horses, and donkeys) are typically bitten on a limb. Goats, sheep, and pigs frequently bite their limbs, head-neck area, belly, and thorax. Dogs are usually bitten on the head, neck, or leg. Poisonous snake bite marks typically reveal distinct puncture wounds from fangs, with or without minor markings from other teeth.

Three toxic snake species, the cobra, krait, and Russell's viper, are common in India. A venomous snakebite is characterized as neurotoxic, myotoxic, hemotoxic, or cytotoxic based on the type of snake involved and the type of venom produced. Cobra and krait venoms are neurotoxic, while viper venom (Russell's viper, saw scaled viper, pit viper) is hemotoxic. Non-poisonous snake bites leave a semicircular pattern of teeth marks. A non-poisonous snake bite does not cause oedema at the bite site, even after many hours.

Symptoms

The severity and type of harm produced by venom vary according to the type of snake, the bite place, and the size of the affected animal.

Symptoms observed in patients following a cobra or krait bite are :

- Puncture wounds at bite site
- Severe pain.
- Localized selling and necrosis.
- Difficulty swallowing or opening eyes.
- Pupillary dilation.
- Dribbling of saliva.
- Symptoms include tremors, flaccid paralysis, and convulsions.
- Death comes from respiratory paralysis caused by depression of the respiratory center and allergies.

Symptoms observed in patients following a bite from a hemototoxic snake

- Swelling is progressive and rising.
- If bitten on a leg, there may be lameness.
- If bitten on the face, asymmetrical swelling can produce dyspnea.
- Bleeding from the biting location. Death occurs as a result of shock.

Diagnosis

Diagnosis of snakebite is difficult in animals.

- On-site witness to snake bite.
- Identified by fang marks in the swelled area and blood seeping from the bite location.
- Symptoms of a hemotoxic snake bite include bleeding at the bite site and swelling on the affected limb.

- A complete blood count, serum chemical profile, and blood clotting time can aid in diagnosis.

In hemotoxic snake bites

- Increased bleeding,
- Increased blood clotting time,
- Thrombocytopenia,
- Leukocytosis, and
- Higher BUN and creatinine levels.

Treatment

The irreversible consequences of venom start shortly after the bite. Thus, aggressive treatment should begin immediately. The primary goal of snakebite treatment is to prevent the spread of venom throughout the body. Pit viper bite therapy consists of treating shock, neutralizing venom, managing blood coagulation, and preventing subsequent bacterial infections.

- Tie two bandages tightly above and below the snake bite site.
- Prevent poison spread by keeping the animal calm and immobilized.
- Avoid using hot or cold compresses as they can cause more tissue injury.
- Polyvalent anti-snake venom. 10-20 cc in 500 ml of 5% dextrose intravenously can save animals' lives.
- Avoid cutting over fang marks or wounds. - Avoid attempting to extract venom through sucking.
- Fluid treatment should be administered.
- Antibiotics such as penicillin and streptomycin should be administered.
- A corticosteroid, such as dexamethasone (2 mg/kg IV), should be administered. It should not be administered to pregnant animals.
- For large animals, haemostat-like carbazochrome salicylate (10 ml IM) should be administered, whereas dogs should receive botropase (1 ml IM/IV).
- Tetanus toxoid should be given, especially to horses.

Scorpion Bite

Each scorpion is venomous. Bite of a scorpion paralyzes the target and kills it. Scorpion venom can kill smaller animals like dogs. Scorpion venom consists of enzyme inhibitors, neurotoxins, and other chemicals. Dogs can be poisoned by scorpions when their venom penetrates their bodies after a sting.

Clinical signs

A scorpion sting can produce symptoms ranging from mild to severe in animals. Several factors determine the range and severity of symptoms, including the patient's physical condition and body mass, the type of scorpion involved and its level of agitation, the amount of venom injected, and the position and depth of the sting.

- Severe discomfort at the biting site.
- Burning feeling at the biting site.
- Weakness.
- Experiencing profuse sweating, difficulty breathing/gasping, pupil dilation, vomiting, diarrhea, and shock-like symptoms within 4-6 hours. After 10 hours, pulmonary edema occurs and blood is vomited. The animals may die within 2-3 days owing to respiratory or cardiac collapse.

Treatment

- To treat a sting, use a blade to make an incision and clean the area with soap and water afterwards.
- Apply ice or cold compress to the affected area.
- Ensure the animal has enough water to consume.
- Provide an antihistamine or corticosteroid.

Spider Bite

Most spiders are venomous.Widow spiders typically bite only when they are accidentally touched. When the bite location is pressed, intense pain occurs. Common symptoms include vomiting, abdominal muscle rigidity, and jelly-like oedema around the bite. There could be escalating motor paralysis. Cardiopulmonary failure may cause death.

Treatment

- If a specialized antivenom (lactrodectus antivenin) is available, animals suspected of serious envenomation should get it. Prior to administration, patients' sensitivity should be evaluated; thereafter, the vial should be diluted with normal saline and slowly infused over 15 minutes. Relief from the symptom is usually given within 30 minutes after administration.
- Muscle relaxants and benzodiazepines, such as diazepam (0.2-0.5 mg/kg BW in dogs, horses, and pigs; 0.05 mg/kg BW in cattle, sheep, and goats, slow IV), can help reduce muscle spasms.

- Atropine is used to prevent salivation.Corticosteroids and hydration therapy are used to treat shock.

Bees Stings

Animals are vulnerable to bee stings when they mistakenly disturb the nest or swarm, which is more common during warm weather when the insects are active.

Clinical signs

- Head-related facial oedema.
- Severe swelling causes dyspnoea.

Treatment

- Remove any stings from the site.
- Clean the area with an alkaline solution.
- Diphenhydramine (1-2 mg/kg IM) is an antihistaminic.
- Corticosteroid (dexamethasone at 0.2 mg/kg, slow IV).
- Neurotonic vitamins B1, B6, and B12 (5-10 ml in large animals and 1-2 ml in small animals, IM).

Lizard Bite

The Indian domestic lizard is not venomous. Bite wounds created by dangerous lizards' top teeth can transmit venom. Animals begin vomiting following poisoning. Shock and death are possible outcomes in severe situations.

Treatment

- Use direct pressure on the wound to halt bleeding.
- Check the wound for lizard teeth.
- Immediately wash the wound thoroughly with running water.
- Apply ice to bite wounds.
- Apply an antiseptic solution to the wound, such as chlorhexidine gluconate, isopropyl alcohol, or povidone-iodine.Antihistaminic and systemic antibiotic treatment are required.

Dog Bites

A dog bite causes significant damage to the skin and soft tissue at the bite site. A dog can bite an animal anywhere on its body. In all cases of dog bites, quick medical attention and post-bite anti-rabies immunizations are required. Dogs have extraordinarily strong teeth and jaws, and the wounds they inflict can cause extensive skin and muscle damage (Fig. 3.1), with some piercing through the chest wall and causing lung collapse. A dog bite can cause deadly intestinal damage.

Each bite wound is believed to be polluted and/or infected. Any bite that tears the skin can introduce germs or other infectious organisms behind the skin's surface, where they can multiply and spread throughout the underlying tissues. If an infected bite wound is not treated, the bacteria might produce a localized abscess or a more extensive tissue infection known as cellulitis, which spreads across the surrounding area.

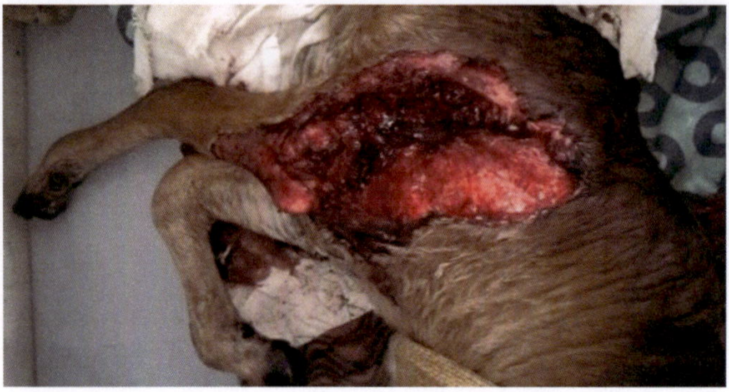

Fig. 3.1. Dog bite wound in a Gir calf showing extensive skin and muscle damage.

Diagnosis

An eyewitness to the dog bite at the incident scene. A veterinarian should check the biting wound.

Treatment

Treatment is determined on the amount of the injury and the location of the wound. If there is a dog owner nearby, inquire about his or her dog's rabies vaccination history.

- Clean the wound with soap and warm water.
- To halt bleeding, gently put a clean cloth over the bite incision.
- To halt bleeding, gently put a clean cloth over the wound.
- Apply antimicrobial ointment to the wound and cover it with a sterile bandage.
- Check the wound for infection.
- Deeply profound bite wounds require surgical closure.
- Administer 1 ml of anti-rabies vaccination (ARV) SC/IM on days 0, 3, 7, 14, 28, and 90. The day of the bite is designated day zero, and ARV should be administered as soon as possible.

References

Ananda K. J., Mohan K., Kamran A and Sharada R (2009). Snake bite in dogs and its successful treatment. Veterinary World, 2(2): 66-67.

Aye K P, Thanachartwet V, Soe C, Desakom V, Thwin K D, Chamnanchanut S, Supaporn T and Sitprija V (2017). Clinical and laboratory parameters associated with acute kidney injury in patients with snakebite envenomation: A prospective observational study from Myanmar. BMC Nephrology 18(92): 1–18.

Bhikane A U, Jadhav R K, Masare P S and Chavhan S G (2020). Clinical, hematobiochemical, and pathological findings and therapeutic management of viperine snake envenomation in zebu cattle. Tropical Animal Health and Production 52: 3425– 37.

Goddard A, Johan P S, Leisewitz A L, Nagel S and Aroch I (2011). Clinicopathologic abnormalities associated with snake envenomation in domestic animals. Veterinary Clinical Pathology 40(3): 282–92.

Menon J C and Joseph J K (2015). Complications of Hemotoxic Snakebite in India. Clinical Toxinology in Asia Pacific and Africa Toxinology, Springer, Dordrecht 2: 209–32.

Sawane CS, Jadhav RK, Bhikane A U, Masare PS, Kushwaha N(2023). Epidemiological, clinical and hematobiochemical studies on hemotoxic snakebite in bovines. Indian Journal of Animal Sciences 93 (1): 23–28.

Scorpion Stings in Animals: Diagnosis and Treatment (2015). Available at https://www.sava.co.za/vetnews/2015/December/VN%20CPD%20December%202015.pdf.

Slagboom J, Kool J, Harrison R A and Casewell N R (2017). Haemotoxic snake venoms: their functional activity, impact on snakebite victims and pharmaceutical promise. British Journal of Haematology 177(6): 947–59.

Textbook of Clinical Veterinary Medicine by MC Sharma, Mahesh Kumar and RD Sharma(2009). Directorate of Information and Publications of Agriculture, ICAR. PP: 552-555.

4

Bleeding

Kumari Chandrakala

Key Points

- Sudden severe bleeding or hemorrhage can cause hemorrhagic shock and death.
- Chronic and or occult bleeding or hemorrhage can cause anemia and even death.
- Common causes of bleeding include trauma, surgical incisions, extreme temperatures, vitamin K deficiency, medicines, and toxins.

Introduction

Bleeding is the extravasation (arterial, venous, or capillary) of blood caused by trauma or a surgical incision.

Classification

External bleeding*-bleeding from the wound or through natural orifices of the body.*

- Bleeding from the nose (epistaxis).
- Hemoptysis (bright red frothy oxygenated blood) refers to bleeding from the nose or respiratory passages.
- Bloody vomiting (hematemesis)
- Melena (partially digested blood): blood in feces.
- Hematuria refers to the presence of blood in urine.

Internal bleeding - occurs on the side of the body and gathers in any natural or newly produced cavity (hematoma).

- Hemorrhage in the pleural cavity-hemopleura.
- Hemorrhage in the peritoneal cavity (hemoperitoneum).
- Hematocele caused by hemorrhage into the testicles' tunica vaginalis.
- Hemorrhage resulting in joint hemarthrosis.

- Hematosalpinx refers to a hemorrhage into the fallopian tube.
- Hemorrhage into the uterus (hemometra).
- Hemorrhage in the extradural part of the spinal cord (hematocolpos).
- Hematomyelia: spinal cord hemorrhage.
- Apoplexy due to brain hemorrhage.
- Pin-point hemorrhage on skin/subcutis- petechiae.
- Ecchymosis is a hmorrhagic patch on the skin or subcutis.

Causes

- Trauma
- Surgical incision
- Nasal granuloma
- Hot summer/ cold winter
- Vit K, vit-C or Ca deficiency
- Tumour

- **Method of controlling bleeding**
- **Irradication of the main source of bleeding**

a) Keep the bleeding component in the rest position.

b) Applying a tourniquet around an extremity, such as the tail, arm, or penis, for not more than 15 minutes.

c) Wrap a tight bandage around the bleeding location on the distal extremity.

d) Thermocautery involves using a red hot iron to stop bleeding from a bigger vessel. Electric thermocautery is now widely available.

e) By using artery forceps.

f) Through crushing or torsion.

g) Ligation is the most effective way to stop bleeding from a vessel.

h) Topical application of adrenaline (causes vasoconstriction).

i) Vitamin K injection (Inj. Kapilin).

j) Administer injectable calcium (calcium boro-gluconate) at a rate of 10-20 ml per large animal.

k) Administration of injectable formalin (38% formaldehyde) in 100 mL of distilled water.

l) Apply gelatin sponge immediately over bleeding spot.

m) Apply liquid tincture Benzoin, ice, and cold water.

n) Inject 250-500 mg of Ethamsylate four times a day intramuscularly or intravenously (cattle, dog, cat).
o) Use Hemocoagulase Inj BOTROPASE at 0.5-1ml (total dosage).
p) Use herbal boluses such as STYPLON VET BOLUS at 1-2 boluses per day.
q) To treat nasal granuloma, use Anthiomaline. For nasal hemorrhage, apply an ice compress to the head or nose.
r) Note: Styptics are injections used to check bleeding.
s) Blood transfusion may be required in cases of severe blood loss.
t) DEXTRANE (200-300/large animal IV)
u) Chromostat injection (10-20 ml/large animal).

References

A Handbook for Veterinary Physician (17Th Revised and Enlarged Edition) SAPRE V. A; Dakshinkar N.P.

Essentials of Veterinary Surgery, 8th Edition, Venugopalan.A,January 2018.

Hand Book of Veterinary Practitioners: Das S.K. Edition: 1st 2005 Rept. 2018.

Handbook of Vet clinician Dr Bhikane A.U and Dr. Kawitkar S.B 1ST JAN 2022.

https://www.msdvetmanual.com/circulatory-system/anemia/hemolytic-anemia-in-animals.

5

Wound

Mamta Mishra

Key Points

- Provide immediate first-aid for wounds.
- For bite wounds, open healing is preferable.
- Silver nanoparticles have antibacterial properties and have been investigated for anticancer applications.

Introduction

Cuts, tears, burns, fractures, and other forms of live tissue injury are all considered wounds. Wounds are typically classified as clean, contaminated, or diseased. Clean wounds are ones that occur in sterile settings, such as surgical incisions. The quantity of germs present distinguishes between contaminated and infected wounds.

Initial Wound Management

The initial step in wound management should be to assess the animal's general stability. Obvious open wounds can divert attention away from more subtle but possibly fatal conditions (such as shock). The general health of the animal influences all areas of care and healing. Some diseases, such as anemia, may impair wound healing by lowering oxygen levels. Malnutrition may also disrupt the healing process. After the initial assessment, the patient should be stable.

Wound irrigation, or lavage, removes both visible and microscopic material. This lowers the risk of infection by reducing the bacterial load. Wound lavage is most effective when administered at the optimum pressure. Low-pressure methods, such as a bulb syringe, are sufficient for clean wounds. Higher pressures are utilized on filthy or infected wounds. A 35-mL syringe and a 19-gauge needle can be used to create a suggested lavage system with a pressure of 48-55 kPa (7-8 psi). Excessive pressure can harm healthy tissue by forcing particles further into it.

To clean a wound, use a syringe to spray a solution onto or into it. Cleaning, also known as debridement, removes dead tissue and foreign material from the wound, which lowers bacterial contamination and helps to avoid infection. Wound lavage has two uses. The optimal lavage fluid should be antibacterial and non-toxic to healing tissues. Saline (0.9% NaCl) solution is the least damaging to healing tissue, although it is not an antiseptic. Surgical scrub agents should be avoided since the detergent components are harmful to tissue. Diluted antiseptics can be used safely.

Chlorhexidine diacetate (0.05%) maintains residual efficacy against a wide range of microorganisms while generating minimal tissue irritation. However, gram-negative bacteria may develop resistance to chlorhexidine. Higher concentrations of chlorhexidine are harmful to healing tissue. Povidone-iodine is an efficient antiseptic; however, it has little residual activity and can be inactivated by purulent material. If the wound is infected, a sample should be taken for bacterial culture and antibiotic susceptibility testing. Antimicrobial treatment should be initiated in all cases of unclean, infected, or punctured wounds. A broad-spectrum bactericidal antibiotic (such as a first-generation cephalosporin) is often suggested pending culture findings. Analgesia is used to relieve pain.

Active bleeding can be managed with direct pressure. In cases of severe arterial bleeding, a pneumatic cuff or pressure wrap should be used instead of a tourniquet; the cuff should be inflated until the hemorrhage is under control. The use of a cuff or pressure wrap can prevent neurovascular problems caused by narrow tourniquets.

Debridement, infection or inflammation control, and moisture balance should all be considered while treating any local wound. Cover the wound with a sterile, lint-free dressing to prevent further contamination or trauma. To reduce bacterial contamination, the time between evaluation and definitive debridement should be kept as short as possible. Following an initial inspection, irrigation, and cleansing, the veterinarian will determine whether to seal the wound or leave it open. Every wound must be evaluated separately. If there is insufficient skin to close the incision or the danger of infection is significant, the wound may remain open.

Debridement

After wound preparation and hair removal, surgical debridement (the removal of non-viable tissue and foreign debris) can take place. Debridement can be conducted non-carefully, removing huge segments of tissue, or more selectively, preserving certain tissues.

Before attempting any debridement, the viability of the skin and nearby tissues should be examined. Skin that is blue-black, leathery, thin, or white is typically not viable. The necrotic tissue should be removed sharply. Debridement can be performed in layers or as one entire portion of tissue (en bloc resection). Tissues of dubious viability or those connected with vital structures like neurovascular bundles should be treated carefully. Staged debridement is recommended in some cases. In addition to sharp dissection, debridement can be autolytic, mechanical (for example, bandage debridement), enzymatic, or biological (maggot treatment).

Selective trimming of live tissue at wound edges (i.e., "freshening the edges") is generally not advised in acute wound management. However, it may improve wound closure when the morphology of the wound renders closure difficult.

Wound Closure

After the initial evaluation, lavage, and debridement, a veterinarian must determine whether to seal the wound or treat it as an open wound. Considerations include the availability of skin for closure, wound location, and the extent of contamination or infection. Although primary closure is the most basic approach to wound management, it should only be utilized in specific instances to minimize wound complications. **Wounds can be closed using sutures, staples, or cyanoacrylate**.

Clean, adequately debrided wounds normally heal without issues. With a primary closure, the layers should be closed individually to reduce "dead space" that could lead to seroma formation. The suture types and patterns employed are determined by the surgeon's preference, the size of the incision, its location, and the animal's size.

Primary closure may not be acceptable for a wound that is severely polluted or infected. As a result, if closure is the goal, it may be postponed until the contamination or illness has been addressed. The wound can be treated as an open wound until it appears healthy. At that point, the wound can be safely closed with little chance of problems. The period between the first debridement and the final closure varies depending on the level of contamination or infection. Wounds that are minimally infected can be closed in 24-72 hours. Largely infected wounds may necessitate longer treatment times.

Secondary closure refers to wounds that are closed more than 5 days after the initial wounding. This means that granulation tissue has formed in the wound prior to closure.

Drains

Drains are used to extract liquids from a wound or body cavity. This keeps the body from "walling off" the fluid, which might cause infection. Drains may be passive or active. Gravity draws the fluid out while using passive drainage techniques. To remove fluid from the wound, active drainage procedures require the use of suction. Extracted fluid can be subjected to laboratory examinations.

Bandages

Bandages help to stop bleeding, keep the wound clean, protect the wound from additional harm, and avoid excessive drying. Bandages come in three layers.

The initial layer of bandage, also known as the dressing, is applied directly to the wound. It could be constructed of gauze or a mesh material that encourages early healing. This layer permits fluid to pass through to the secondary layer of the bandage while also protecting tissue from drying out. Removing the bandages can be painful, but it helps debride and clean the tissue. Wet-to-dry bandages are created from moistened gauze that is applied directly to the wound. They can sometimes be uncomfortable to remove, but they dry the tissue more slowly than dry bandages.

The second layer of a bandage helps absorb fluid, pad the wound, and support or immobilize the limb.

This layer is typically made of cast padding or roll cotton. The third layer applies pressure to the wound, keeps the inner layers in place, and protects them from the environment. Typically, this layer consists of adhesive tape or elastic wrap.

Open wound management

Wounds left untreated are typically treated with frequent bandaging and debridement. Wet-to-dry dressings are commonly utilized. These dressings help to clean the wound with each bandage change. In the early phases of recovery, the bandage may need to be changed up to twice a day. Dry, nonstick dressings are applied once the wound has healed. A wound can be closed after it has been treated for some time. This is frequent when an illness exists but is successfully treated with antibiotics. Such wounds can be closed after 24 to 72 hours, or more (Fig. 5.1).

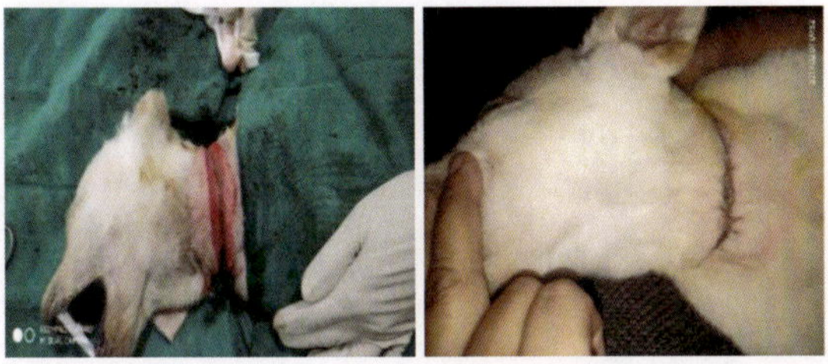

Fig. 5.1. An open wound at the neck of a dog caused by kite string (Days 0 and 14)

Wounds can be closed using sutures, staples, or surgical adhesive. Sometimes numerous levels of closure are required. For example, a deep layer of sutures may be required to hold torn muscles together, as well as an exterior layer of sutures to close the skin over them.

Surgical management

Sometimes a wound necessitates surgical intervention. Different sorts of wounds necessitate different surgical approaches. To close a wound, skin flaps may be stretched over it. Muscle flaps are also utilized to treat deep wounds. Sometimes skin (or muscle) from other locations, or grafts, are extracted and surgically joined to cover a wound; thus, the nearest veterinary hospital should be visited.

Many topical medications are used to treat wounds. These could be meant to encourage natural wound closure, prevent infection, or alleviate discomfort. various topical medications (used for various purposes) may impede wound healing. When determining the best course of action, your veterinarian will weigh the potential risks and advantages.

Management of Specific Wounds

Cuts and Tears (Lacerations)

Lacerations are wounds or tears in the skin. Uncomplicated simple lacerations occur when there is no deep tissue involvement or other severe issues. Such incisions are normally treated with complete closure; however, this may not be possible if the wound is unclean or infected. Deep cuts can be treated similarly to simple ones, depending on the severity of the damage. Muscles, tendons, and other tissues must be repaired before a wound can be closed. Uncomplicated lacerations are usually treated with full closure if they are not severely infected.

Prior to closure, the wound should be completely lavaged and debrided as needed. If tension exists on the wound borders, it should be released using tension-relieving suture methods, sliding tissue flaps, or grafts. Deep lacerations may be treated using the same methods, depending on the severity of the damage. Prior to closure, any underlying structures (such as muscles, tendons, and blood vessels) must be repaired. If a laceration is severely polluted with debris, primary wound closure may be unnecessary. Contaminated wounds can be closed with drains or managed as open wounds.

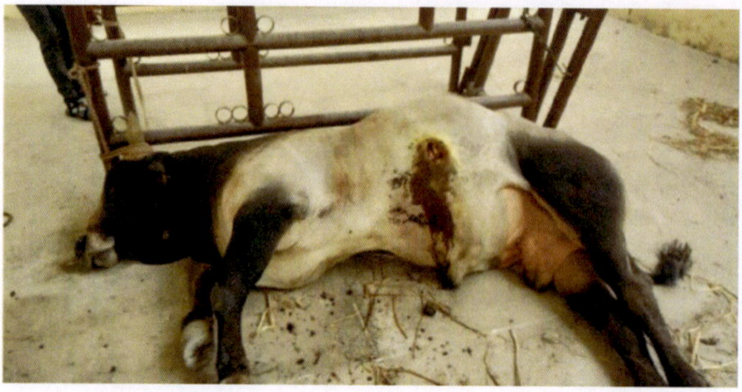

Fig. 5.2. Open wound management of a contaminated wound in a bull.

Bite Wounds

Bite wounds are a leading cause of injury, particularly in free-ranging animals.

Cat bites are small, piercing wounds that frequently develop infection and require treatment as an abscess, including culture, debridement, antibiotics, and wound drainage.

Dog bites have a more diverse presentation. Because dog bite injuries are slashing in nature, the majority of the tissue damage occurs beneath the wound's surface. Although just minor puncture marks or bruising appear on the surface, ribs may be fractured or internal organs severely wounded.

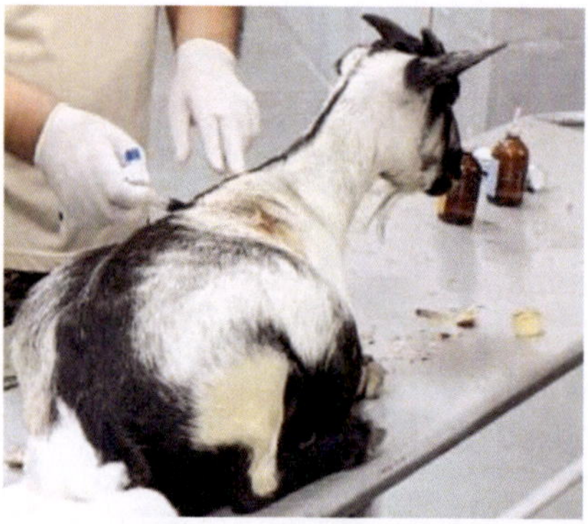

Fig. 5.3. Antiseptic dressing of dog bite wounds in a goat.

Before beginning definitive wound care, the patient should have been properly assessed and stabilized. Before deciding on a repair, the wound should be surgically stretched to allow for a comprehensive evaluation and determination of its extent. Debridement might be conducted following a thorough evaluation. Complete wound closure is rarely indicated unless en bloc debridement is performed since the sites are polluted. Depending on the severity of the injury, drainage, delayed closure, or second intention can all be used to close the wound; however, dog bite wounds cannot.

De-gloving injuries

De-gloving injuries involve the shearing or tearing of the skin. De-gloving injuries can develop on the legs, torso, and paws. Skin loss is frequently substantial, with deeper tissues also affected. Animals injured by cars or caught under the hood frequently suffer de-gloving injuries (Fig. 5.4). Sometimes the skin is not fully removed. It stays linked to the surrounding skin but not to the tissues beneath it. The skin is loose, often damaged, and delicate. It may perish later since it does not have a blood supply.

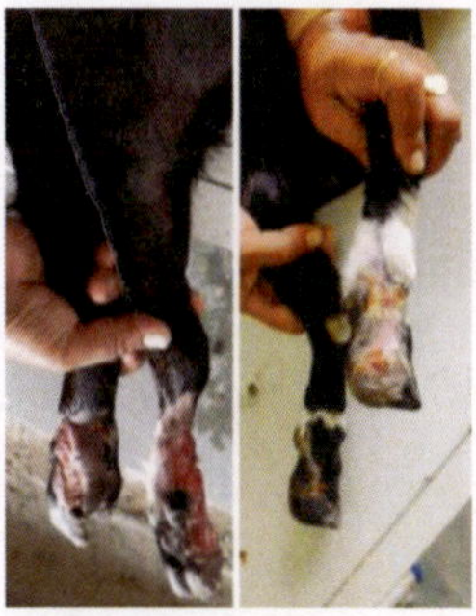

Fig. 5.4. Accidental degloving injury of forelimbs in a goat.

All dead skin and other tissue must be removed. Tissue that can be recoverd is typically saved. Infection is a serious consequence, and avoiding infection is the primary goal of treatment. De-gloving injuries often necessitate significant and recurrent debridement. Early wound debridement may make it difficult to distinguish between viable and nonviable tissue. An attempt should be made to save tissue whose viability is uncertain. Any necrotic tissue can be removed with further debridement.

Gunshot injuries

The majority of the damage in gunshot injuries is hidden since the wounds are usually deep. Gunshot wounds are also polluted because the bullet or pellet carries skin, hair, and debris into the wound. If the bullet escapes the body, it will leave a larger wound than it entered. High-speed bullets send shock waves through surrounding tissue and organs, resulting in blunt-force injuries.

Surgery is required to assess the extent of damage caused by a gunshot wound. Organ and deep tissue damage are potentially fatal. Fractures are common and may necessitate further therapy or surgery.

Pressure Wounds

Pressure wounds, also known as decubital ulcers, are caused by sustained pressure on a specific area of skin. When tissues do not receive enough blood or oxygen, they begin to die. Pressure wounds are extremely difficult to treat and are best avoided.Paraplegia, tetraplegia, inappropriate coaptation, and immobility are all risk factors for pressure sores.

Preventive strategies include changing the animal's position periodically, ensuring enough feed and sanitation, and providing a well-padded bed. If pressure wounds are minor or discovered early, cleaning and bandaging may be sufficient to avoid additional harm. More severe wounds necessitate intensive surgical treatment. Following debridement and the formation of a granulation bed, an advancement flap or pedicle graft may be necessary for closure.

Traditional therapeutics for wound management

Sugar has been used as a cheap wound dressing for over three centuries to prevent odor and infection. Sugar's use is based on its high osmolality, which sucks fluid out of the wound while inhibiting bacterial development. Sugar also aids in the removal of necrotic tissue while protecting viable tissue.

To absorb fluid taken from the wound, a 1 cm thick coating of granulated sugar is placed in the wound cavity and covered with a thick covering. The sugar dressing should be changed once a day or anytime there is strikethrough (fluid soaking from the wound to the bandage surface). During the bandage change, liberally rinse the wound with warm saline (0.9% NaCl) or tap water.

Honey has also been used as a wound treatment for millennia. Honey's high osmolality, low pH, and hydrogen peroxide activity all contribute to its positive benefits. However, methyl-glyoxal is the primary contributor to honey's antibacterial properties. Honey can be applied directly to the wound or soaked into a contact dressing. The use of honey should be restricted to the inflammatory phase. Once a granulation bed has formed, continuing usage may dehydrate the area or traumatize the healing tissue during removal.

Silver has been utilized as a topical agent in various formulations for hundreds of years. Silver is accessible in creams (silver sulfadiazine) or imbedded in dressings. Silver nanoparticles have antibacterial properties and have also been investigated for anticancer applications. Silver is recommended for use during the inflammatory stage of wound healing. While its mechanism is unknown, it is bactericidal and may promote angiogenesis and reduce wound scarring.

Zinc-containing antibiotics (such as bacitracin-zinc) may promote wound healing by contributing zinc to the wound bed. Zinc has been demonstrated to possess antibacterial and anti-inflammatory effects.Given the restricted ability of topical antibiotics to permeate deeper tissues, systemic antibiotics are recommended.

Enzymatic agents (typically found in ointment formulations) are proteolytic chemicals that liquefy necrotic tissue. These agents are utilized during the inflammatory stage of healing. They do not induce the discomfort associated with surgery, and their usage is recommended in situations where surgical debridement may be damaging to long-term function.

Medicinal maggots are utilized in the inflammatory stage of wound healing to eliminate necrotic tissue and detritus. The common green bottle fly (Lucilia sericata) is utilized to produce medical-grade maggots. The maggots remove necrotic tissue by secreting proteolytic enzymes that liquefy the waste. Maggots also have a positive impact by consuming microorganisms. Finally, certain of the secretions may prevent biofilm development. Maggot therapy may be contraindicated in dry wounds, and it should not be used as the primary treatment in infected patients.

References

Bellah JR and Williams JM (1999). Wound closure options and decision making: Fowler D. Williams J.M. Manual of canine and feline wound management and reconstruction. British Small Animal Veterinary Association, Cheltenham (UK): 25-36

Hendrix CM (1991). Facultative myiasis in dogs and cats. Compend Contin Educ Pract Vet.; 13: 86-94

Lee AH., Swaim SF., McGuire JA (1987). Effects if nonadherent dressing materials on the healing of open wounds in dogs. J Am Vet Med Assoc.; 190: 416-422

Singh J., Singh S., and Tyagi, RPS (2019). Wound Healing and Repair: Ruminant Surgery: A Textbook of the Surgical Diseases of Cattle, Buffaloes, Camels, Sheep and Goats [CBS Publishers & Distributors]: pp 105-120

Slatter DH. (2003). Wound repair and specific tissue responses to injury: Textbook of Small Animal Surgery [Saunders], Vol 1: 66-86

Swaim SF and Henderson RA (1997). Wound management: Swaim S.F. Henderson R.A. Small animal wound management. 2nd edition. Williams & Wilkins, Baltimore (MD): 13-51

Swaim SF., Riddell KP and McGuire JA (1992) Effects of topical medications on the healing of open pad wounds in dogs. J Am Anim Hosp Assoc.; 28: 499-502

6

Burn

Kumari Chandrakala

Key Points

- Burns are injuries caused by hot solids or flames.
- Scalds are injuries caused by liquids or steam.

Type of burn	1° burn	2° burn (most painful)	3° burn
Tissue layer involved	Epidermis	Epidermis + dermis	Epidermis + dermis+ S/C fat, muscle/other deeper parts
Physical symptoms	Diffuse swelling/ vesicle formation	Blister formation	Skin appears brownish black and leathery
Healing time	10 days	3-4week	3-4week or more

> 4% burn causes shock.

> 50% burn poor prognosis.

Treatment

Dehydration/Shock: NSS I/V

Petroleum jelly or liquid paraffin serves as an emollient (moisturizer).

Calamine lotion is an astringent (vasoconstriction) and cleanser.

Local analgesics (reduces burning feeling and pain): 2% lignocaine gel.

Antiseptic ointment and systemic antibiotics.

Acidic solution burns are treated with an alkaline solution (sodium bicarbonate) and plenty of plain water.

Alkaline solution burns are treated with an acidic solution (vinegar) and plenty of plain water.

7

Frostbite

Anand Mohan

Key Points

- Frostbite occurs when exposed to freezing temperatures. Animals that are weak and malnourished are more likely to be injured.
- It is a prevalent condition throughout the winter, particularly in animals who do not have shelter or have inadequate protection to protect them from the cold.
- Excessive cold can harm skin and subcutaneous tissue. In severe circumstances, injuries may be irreversible.

Introduction

Frostbite, also known as freezing cold damage, is caused by prolonged exposure to temperatures below 0° C. Exposure to freezing temperatures causes excessive heat loss, disrupting the body's heat balance and resulting in systemic or local acute freezing injury. Frost bites cause superficial tissue injury, but in extreme cases, gangrene develops in the joint or synovial sheath, and the animal dies from toxemia. However, all animal species are susceptible. It occurs rarely in healthy and well-nourished animals. Animals that have lost their coats or are malnourished are particularly vulnerable to harm. Prolonged exposure to colder temperatures increases the risk of frostbite and the severity of the injury. In the majority of cases, frostbite occurs in animals that are left in winter.

Aetiology

Frostbite occurs when the skin is exposed to freezing temperatures for an extended period of time. The nose, ears, scrotum, snout, tail, teats, extremities, comb, and wattles are particularly vulnerable. Newborn calves and children born in cold, windy environments (below 0°C) are more susceptible to frostbite. The damage occurs more frequently in weak calves or when peripheral circulation is impeded due to diarrhea and dehydration. Animals exposed to extremely low temperatures for an extended period of time, particularly those not fed healthy food, will experience a decline in body temperature due to heat loss. Muscles become stiff. Animals are hesitant to move because of muscle stiffness, and when forced to move, they do so slowly. Immobility further reduces the temperature.

A break in the integument allows cold to damage the tissue beneath the skin. It produces dermatitis in varying degrees. Gangrene can sometimes progress to gangrenous dermatitis. The gangrene may extend to a joint or an essential synovial sheath, and the toxicity may be severe enough to kill the animal. When the body temperature drops below 70° F, the heartbeat stops.

Clinical findings

Frost bite intensity can range from brief tissue chilling to freezing and necrosis of a section of the tissue.

In mild frost bites -

- The skin initially appears pale and bloodless, followed by acute redness, heat, severe discomfort, and swelling.
- Sensory loss during palpation.
- The affected part becomes chilly or brittle.
- Hair loss from the afflicted area.
- Within a few days, the epidermis peels and irritation decreases.

If the heat is removed at this point, the condition will return to normal.

When tissues are exposed to temperatures below 0°C for an extended period of time, they suffer vessel wall damage and tissue inflammation. The epidermis shows redness, necrosis, and blister formation, followed by desquamation. When the temperature drops below freezing, blood and lymph circulation stop, and the part succumbs to necrosis with gangrene.

In severe situations, the affected area becomes bloated and painful, resulting in necrosis. The intensity of the exposure and subsequent cellular damage determine whether the effects are reversible or irreversible.

- Skin color ranges from dark blue to black.
- Patches of skin are damaged, creating a distinct line between the affected and normal areas.
- Dead skin sheds over the course of few days or weeks, resulting in a rough surface.
- Common symptoms in calves include a rusty muzzle, devitalized ear tips and tail ends, and chilly hind feet.
- When a calf lies down, its forefeet are positioned beneath the body, providing warmth and protection from cold.

- Calf's often place their front feet under their body to defend against cold.
- Devitalized tissue, including hooves, begins to slough after a few days or weeks, leading to the calf's refusal to stand.
- A secondary bacterial infection worsens the disease, resulting in pus formation and a bad odor. It slows the healing process and necessitates additional attention.

Diagnosis

A history of exposure to freezing temperatures and clinical indications are sufficient to diagnose frost bite.

Treatment

Frostbite must be treated immediately. To prevent further harm, cover the exposed region. Rewarming is the initial stage of treatment. There are some crucial things to remember when treating frostbite.

- Do not use hot water to warm frostbitten areas, as it can worsen the damage.
- Avoid applying direct heat to sensitive areas, such as with a hair dryer or heating pad.
- Avoid massaging or rubbing the affected regions while they are warming up.
- Gently and quickly defrost frozen tissue in warm water at 100.2 ° to 111.1 ° F (38-44 °C) to avoid refreezing.
- To prevent freezing, heating should be continuous.
- To defrost frozen parts, apply a lukewarm antiseptic lotion. Tissue thawing is unpleasant, so painkillers should be administered. Slow thawing is less painful than quick thawing, but tissue damage is far greater.
- Apply antiseptic to prevent septic problems when there is a breach in the surface. If there is a break on the skin's surface, an antiseptic solution combining turpentine, ammonia, and chloroform (one part each in six parts of a mixed oil basis) is used.
- Hot applications might cause vessel rupture; therefore, avoid using them.
- Leave the wounded area exposed while healing, and avoid using occlusive dressings.

- Premature debridement should be avoided since more tissues may be important than is apparent.
- High-calorie and protein-rich diets, together with vitamin A supplementation, are advantageous.

If an animal has been exposed to a severe cold, it should not be quickly moved to a heated environment or given a hot bath. This could lead to the animal's death owing to thrombosis, embolism, or internal organ congestion.

Access to shelter, as well as proper hydration and nourishment, can help prevent frostbite.

References

Diterich, R.A (1983). Cold Injury. In: Current Veterinary Therapy. 8th edition, Kirk, R.W. (Ed.) W.B. Saunders Co., Philadelphia. PP: 187-189.

Roche-Nagle G, Murphy D, Collins A and Sheehan S (2008). Frostbite: management options. Eur J Emerg Med. 15(3): 173-175.

Sudan, N.A. and Bhawal, M.S. (2009). Miscellaneous diseases conditions. In: Textbook of Veterinary Medicine. Sharma, MC., Mahesh Kumar and Sharma, R.D. (Ed.), ICAR, Krishi Anusandhan Bhavan, Pusa, New Delhi. PP: 590-592.

8

Electrocution

Mamta Mishra

Key Points

- Animals can experience varying levels of electric shock. Lightning typically kills animals instantaneously and causes them to fall to the ground without struggle.Most electric shock deaths are caused by cardiac or respiratory arrest.
- Animals often recover from minutes to several hours, rarely going unconscious. Residual nervous system effects, including sadness, paraplegia, and increased cutaneous sensitivity to painless stimuli, can last for days, weeks, or even months.

Introduction

Lightning strikes, broken transmission lines, malfunctioning electrical circuits, or an animal chewing on an electrical cable can all cause an animal to be injured or killed by high-voltage electrical currents. Lightning strikes are seasonal and occur in thunderstorm-prone regions. Caution should always be maintained when investigating probable electrocution situations because the source of the electrification, such as broken transmission wires, may still be present.

Factors causing increased incidence

Some tree species are more susceptible to lightning strikes than others, notably hardwoods such as oaks and tall trees with extensively scattered root systems directly beneath the ground. When such roots become electric, a vast area of the earth is charged, particularly if the ground is already humid. A shallow pool of water can become electrified when charged roots pass beneath it. A building, fence, or body of water can be electrified by falling or dangling transmission lines.

Clinical findings

The severity of the injury is determined by the type of current, its passage through the body, as well as the volume and length of the current flow. Symptoms vary depending on the amount of voltage to which the animal is exposed. A range of shocks may occur. If an animal is exposed to high voltage, it may die without a struggle. Singing and burning are likely to happen.

Animals become unconscious and struggle after being exposed to low voltages. After gaining consciousness, the animal may recover normally or exhibit sadness, blindness, posterior paralysis, paraplegia, monoplegia, and cutaneous hyperesthesia. Burn lesions start out dry, then develop hyperaemia and oedema during the next 36 hours. Ulcers caused by necrotic tissue sloughing heal gradually.

Necropsy findings

Rigor mortis develops and soon kills animals who are electrocuted. Petechiae on the serous membranes, pulmonary edema, right ventricle engorgement, blood vessel rupture, and thrombosis are all obvious. Linear singe marks are typically found on the medial side of the legs. Capillary congestion and an arboreal pattern are visible on the dermal side of the skin, indicating lightning strokes. Massive hemorrhage and cerebral disorganization. Rumen distension, delayed clotting, linear tracheal hemorrhage, and all other viscera are congested; petechiae and ecchymoses may appear in numerous organs.

Diagnosis

The existence of trees, buildings, fences, and live hanging wires at the location where the animals were discovered, as well as the history of recent storms and lightning, all contribute to the diagnosis. A differential diagnosis of nitrite-nitrate poisoning, black leg syndrome, and tympany should be made.

Treatment

Both lightning strikes and electrocution are true emergencies that necessitate prompt attention from a veterinarian. When a pet chews on an electrical cord, the effects of electrocution may not be immediately apparent, but shock symptoms and other difficulties may develop later. Animals that survive require both supportive and symptomatic therapy.

Depending on the type of trauma or injury sustained, the patient may need cervical or spinal immobilization. A primary assessment should be undertaken as soon as feasible to evaluate severe injuries (e.g., pneumothorax, fractures). Following the primary examination, any patient with substantial burns or suspected rhabdomyolysis (myoglobinuria) should get fluid resuscitation (with a target urine output of 0.5 to 1 mL/kg/h). If more diuresis is required, use an osmotic diuretic (mannitol), a loop diuretic (furosemide), or urine alkalization (with sodium bicarbonate titration).

Treatment is primarily supportive and symptomatic. In unconscious animals, artificial breathing and central nervous system stimulants should be administered. Large animals should receive epinephrine (1:10000) at 0.01 mg/kg IV, chlorpheniramine maleate at 20 mg/kg IM, and dexamethasone at 2 mg/kg, as well as hydration therapy with 5% dextrose and normal saline at 90 ml/kg BW IV.

Antibiotics should be administered twice a day to treat subsequent bacterial infections. The use of NSAIDS (flunixin meglumine, ketoprofen, meloxicam, or tolfenamic acid) is advised. To overcome concurrent hypokalaemia and hypocalcaemia, intravenous calcium and magnesium infusions, as well as potassium chloride, should be administered carefully.

References

Schulze, C., Peters,M., Baumgartner, W., and Wohlsein, P. (2016). Electrical Injuries in Animals: Causes, Pathogenesis, and Morphological Findings. Veterinary Pathology. 53. 10.1177/0300985816643371.

Sudan, N.A. and Bhawal, M.S. (2009). Miscellaneous diseases conditions. In: Textbook of Veterinary Medicine. Sharma, MC., Mahesh Kumar and Sharma, R.D. (Ed.), ICAR, Krishi Anusandhan Bhavan, Pusa, New Delhi, pp: 599-601.

The Merck veterinary manual. Whitehouse Station, NJ :Merck& Co., Inc.

Zemaitis, MR., Foris, LA., Lopez, RA., Huecker MR. (2023). Electrical Injuries. [Updated 2023 Jul 17]. In: StatPearls [Internet]. Treasure Island (FL): StatPearls Publishing; 2024 Jan-. Available from: https://www.ncbi.nlm.nih.gov/books/NBK448087.

9

Hyperthermia

Safeeda Sultana Begum

Key Points

- Physical cooling is more effective in managing hyperthermia.
- Heat stroke occurs when the cause is solely physical.

Introduction

Hyperthermia is an unusually high body temperature (also known as overheating) caused by the body absorbing or producing more heat than it can discharge. Simply said, it is the increase in temperature above the critical point. Heat stroke is most common in animals when they lose control of their body temperature.

Etiology

Animal hyperthermia is typically caused by high ambient or surrounding conditions in which the animal's body is unable to remove heat properly, resulting in a constant rise in body temperature. Examples include animals being restricted to a heat source due to tethering, animals being left tethered in full sunlight during peak summer, or in animal buildings with limited air circulation during peak summer and the most common incident being a fire in an animal house or building. Severe physical exercise in high humidity is another key cause of hyperthermia in animals.

Infections with agents such as bacteria or viruses also induce a fever, which can reach extremely high temperatures. However, hyperthermia plays a minor role in the genesis of infectious agents. Hyperthermia can also be caused by toxicity from drugs such as hops, high thyroid hormone levels, or medications that cause seizures. Malignant hyperthermia is an uncommon reaction to anesthesia or other medicines in which muscles tense and break down, resulting in an elevated body temperature. Porcine stress syndrome causes malignant hyperthermia, which is also seen in horses on rare occasions.

In addition to these, genetics, spontaneous hemorrhage in the hypothalamus (the body's thermoregulatory center; neurogenic hyperthermia), poisoning with specific drugs (levamisole and dinitrophenols) or plants, certain mycotoxins (Clavicepspurpurea, Acremonium coenophialum; cause of epidemic hyperthermia), dehydration (insufficient fluid to accommodate heat loss by evaporation), and so on all cause hyperthermia in various animal species.

Clinical findings

The animal's rectal temperature rises 3 to 4 degrees Celsius (4 to 7 degrees Fahrenheit) above normal. In the early stages, there is an increase in heart and respiratory rates, as well as a weak pulse with a large amplitude, sweating, and salivation, followed by a significant lack of sweat. The animal becomes restless at first, then dulls and prefers to lie down. As the temperature rises, the animal becomes thirsty and exhibits severe irregularities in breathing, pulse, and heart rate, which are frequently followed by collapse, convulsions, and ultimate coma. Most occurrences end in death, and in pregnant animals, prolonged heat may result in abortion.

Diagnosis

A diagnosis can be made using history (particularly the history of the animal environment), clinical findings, and symptoms. The animal's state, such as dull, depressed, dehydrated, dry mucous membrane, dry coat, and so on, might also indicate hyperthermia. In fever, the temperature rarely exceeds 106oF, although in hyperthermia it usually does. Simple hyperthermia should be distinguished from fever and septicemia. Clinically, there may be little distinction between them. Physical examination of a dog reveals dry and hyperaemic mucous membranes, as well as shortened capillary filling time as a result of peripheral vasodilation.

Treatment

In the case of hyperthermic animals exposed to high air temperatures, an adequate supply of drinking water (with or without electrolytes), shade, and good air movement (for effective evaporative cooling) is critical. Fluids, such as normal saline or 5% dextrose, should be administered intravenously. Cold treatments, such as immersion spraying, rectal enema, or cold packs, are also beneficial. Place the injured animal in the shade, pour cold water along the midline of the back (so that the coats are saturated), and monitor the rectal temperature often during this procedure so that water application can be discontinued when the temperature returns to normal.

Severely hyperthermic animals should be given an oxygen-enriched mixture as well as a significant dosage of isotonic or polyionic crystalloid fluid (50 ml/kg body weight in domestic animals and 10 to 20 ml/kg in dogs), such as lactated Ringer's solution or acetated Ringer's solution. In most situations, shade and appropriate cool water, as well as the use of antipyretic and tranquilizing medications (if necessary during conditions of high warmth and humidity combined with confinement), are recommended. The specific and highly successful treatment for malignant hyperthermia is intravenous dantrolene (2.5-10.0 mg/kg body weight).

Antipyretic and non-steroidal anti-inflammatory medicines (NSAIDs) are contraindicated in the care of hospitalized patients because the former's mode of action does not reduce the temperature of hyperthermic patients, functioning solely in the thermoregulatory center to regulate fever. NSAIDs can reduce renal perfusion and increase the risk of gastrointestinal ulcers.

Further management aspects include supplying fans or coolers, shading, water sprinklers, altering the quantity of ration, timing of feeding ration (feeding the larger lot in the cooler evening hours), reducing handling during stressful periods, and so on. If such an etiology is suspected, supportive treatment may include the provision of appropriate glucose and protein, as well as the use of tranquilizing medications to minimize excessive activity in animals. Chlorpromazine has been demonstrated to greatly boost the survival rate of pigs under heat and humidity stress.

References

A text book of the diseases of cattle, sheep, pigs, goats and horses by Radostits O. M., Gay C. C., Blood D. C. and Hinchcliff K.W., 10th edition, Saunders Publication.

Gabriela Goncalves Caldas, Daianne Oliveira Barbosa da Silva and Durval Barauna Junior. (2022). Heat stroke in dogs: Literature review. Veterinarni Medicina, 67(07): 354–364.

10

Hypothermia

Neelam Kushwaha

Key Points

- Hypothermia occurs when an individual's body temperature drops below its critical level.
- Excessive heat loss or inadequate thermoregulation can lead to this condition.
- It can be minor or severe. Mild hypothermia is harmless, while moderate to severe hypothermia is an emergency.

Introduction

Hypothermia is a general systemic state characterized by a disturbance in thermoregulation followed by a drop in body temperature below a crucial threshold. It occurs when heat loss surpasses heat generation. It affects all animals, but newborns, such as piglets, pups, calves, and children, are most vulnerable, especially those born in cold weather and whose moms are unable to lick them dry. This syndrome is referred to as neonatal hypothermia. In newborn animals, activity to control body temperature is low. A quick decline in body temperature in a previously feverish animal indicates a negative prognosis. The diagnosis of hypothermia is made by taking the patient's body temperature. If hypothermia is not treated, it leads to mortality, particularly in neonates.

Etiology

It can be caused by greater heat loss, reduced heat production, or impaired thermoregulation.

Excessive heat loss can occur due to the following:

- Low metabolic activity can lead to heat loss at extreme cold air temperatures.
- Muscular tone and peripheral vasoconstriction are insufficient to compensate.

- Infusion of a cold solution.
- Lie on a chilly, uninsulated surface.
- Induced vasodilation.
- Hyperthermia is treated vigorously or exposed to cold temperatures.
- Possible causes of decreased heat output include reduced muscle tone, such as in parturient paresis.
- Acute ruminal impaction.
- Anesthetic medicines cause depression via the hypothalamic thermostatic system.
- Impaired thermoregulation can occur due to CNS illnesses such as trauma, neoplasia, or edema, as well as endogenous toxemia.

Factors which augments hypothermia are:

Humidity in the air: Because humid air conducts heat more effectively, it swiftly cools the body.

Air movement: Air movement increases cooling intensity.

Animal age: Newborns such as piglets, puppies, calves, and children suffer hypothermia when born in cold weather because their moms are unable to lick them dry. In newborn animals, activity to control body temperature is low. Similarly, when animals age, their vital capacity falls.

Body condition: Emaciated and malnourished animals are more susceptible to hypothermia than healthy and obese animals.

Medicines: Many narcotic medicines produce an increase in heat loss from the body by dilating superficial blood vessels. A rush of blood to the body's surface is beneficial for cooling since it increases heat loss.

Management practices: In sheep, hypothermia may be a key contributor to post-shearing mortality, especially if body weight plummeted immediately before shearing.

Calves, lambs, and foals can all have neonatal hypothermia. This is caused by extreme cold weather. Neonates are unable to maintain normal body temperatures for the first few hours following birth.

Clinical signs

Hypothermia can range from mild to severe. Mild hypothermia (over 36°C) is harmless and does not necessitate lengthy rewarming methods. Emergency treatment is required for moderate (above 30°C) to severe (below 30°C) hypothermia. The clinical indications of hypothermia are:

- Reduced body temperature (<37 °C)
- Weakness, decreased activity
- Shivering
- Cold extremities (ears, legs, feet, paws)
- Muscle stiffness
- Varying degrees of shock
- Weak pulse and collapse of major veins
- Oral mucous membrane -cool with a lack of saliva
- Pale gums

Prolonged severe hypothermia can result in metabolic acidosis, atrial arrhythmias, ventricular arrhythmias, hypokalaemia, hyponatremia, increased blood viscosity, impaired myocardial function, coagulopathies, hyperglycemias, insulin resistance, hepatic glycogen depletion, and impaired gluconeogenesis, all of which lead to hypoglycemia and cold diuresis.

Neonatal hypothermia in piglets:

- Huddling together
- Lack of sucking drive
- Lethargic, recumbent, and death

Diagnosis

A patient's body temperature is used to diagnose hypothermia. Rectal thermometers provide the most accurate measurements.Clinical indicators aid in the diagnosis.

Upon necropsy: A lack of milk in the stomach in babies with hypothermia.

Treatment

Management of hypothermic patient can be done by:

i. Passive rewarming treatments involve drying the patient's body surfaces and wrapping them in blankets.

ii. Active rewarming methods include heating blankets, infrared heat lamps, warm water baths, electric floor heaters, and hot water bottles.

iii. Active core rewarming procedures involve administering warmed intravenous fluid and flushing the open body cavity, stomach, or rectum with lukewarm sterile isotonic polyionic fluid.

Passive rewarming strategies are only effective in mild to moderate hypothermia, where the patient can generate heat through metabolism or shivering. It is typically harmless, but prolonged use exposes the patient to the harmful effects of hypothermia.

Moderate to severe hypothermia needs external active rewarming treatments. Electric heating blankets and hot water bottles should be used with caution because they can burn the skin if left too hot. If bottles are going to come into contact with skin, the water should not be warmer than 42 °C. In addition, infrared heat lamps are used to warm hypothermic patients. The recommended distance between the lamp and the animal is 75 cm to avoid excessive tissue drying.

Active core rewarming procedures lessen the danger of vascular collapse associated with surface rewarming methods. The amount of fluid that can be safely provided is a limitation when warming a patient via intravenous infusion of warmed fluids (dextrose 5-10%). Fluid supplied should not be heated above 42 degrees Celsius.

Corticosteroids like dexamethasone (except in pregnant animals) and isoflupredone acetate (safe in pregnant animals) can be administered to avoid shock.

Hypothermic new born piglets can be managed by -

- To treat affected piglets, keep them in a warm box, use a heater for rewarming, and administer dextrose intraperitoneally (15 ml 5% glucose solution every 4-6 hours) or orally via stomach tube at a minimum temperature of 30-35°C.

Piglets are fed colostrum and dried manually.

Reference

Textbook of Clinical Veterinary Medicine by MC Sharma, Mahesh Kumar and RD Sharma, Directorate of Information and Publications of Agriculture, ICAR., January 2009. A text book of the diseases of cattle, sheep, pigs, goats and horses by Rodostis O. M., Gay C. C., Blood D. C. and Hinchcliff K.W., 10thedition, Saunders Publication.

11

Drowning

Neelam Kushwaha

Key Points

- Drowning is a common cause of accidental death in animals.
- Submersion in water or other fluids prevents atmospheric air from reaching the lungs.
- To diagnose drowning, trustworthy witnesses and a history of drowning at the accident location are required.

Introduction

Drowning or immersion is a type of asphyxial death caused by a body being submerged in water or another fluid medium and preventing atmospheric air from reaching the lungs. Drowning isn't always fatal. When a drowning causes death, it is known as a fatal drowning. Complete submersion is not required for lethal drowning; simply submerging the nose and mouth is sufficient. Drowning is a difficult process. It comprises liquid aspiration, struggle, involuntary movements, dyspnea, and cardiovascular responses. Drowning ultimately leads to hypoxia and death.

Aetiology

Animals rarely drown because they are natural swimmers. Drowning in animals is caused by a variety of events, including falling into bodies of water from which they cannot escape, mishaps while swimming, seizures or other neurological dysfunctions that make swimming difficult, or deliberate submersion by a person. It can occur during natural disasters such as cyclones and floods. In such cases, multiple animals are impacted at once. Animals may become trapped while crossing a stream of water, which causes it to occur.

Pathogenesis

There are two sorts of drownings: conventional and unusual. Wet drowning, also known as wet drowning, is an obstruction of the airways and lungs caused by the inhalation of water or any fluid. When water is breathed and reaches the lungs, the odds of survival decrease. The volume of fresh or salt water aspirated has an inverse relationship with survival time.

Typical drowning can occur as

a) Fresh water drowning

b) Sea water drowning

If an animal drowns in fresh water, a large amount of water enters (hypotonic) the lungs and is quickly absorbed into the bloodstream, resulting in hypervolemia. Hypervolemia causes haemodilution of erythrocytes, which leads to hemolysis. Ventricular fibrillation can develop from anoxia produced by hemoglobin deficiency in RBCs. Within 3 minutes, aspirated fresh water reaches the circulation of dogs. During freshwater immersion, the lungs can absorb up to 10% of the body weight in water.

If a person drowns in sea water, the hypertonic nature of the water causes rapid salt absorption into the circulation and effusion of water from the blood, resulting in haemoconcentration and pulmonary oedema due to water entering the alveoli, which leads to circulatory shock and cardiac arrest. The death rate from aspiration of salt water is higher than that of fresh water.

Atypical drowning occurs when there is little to no water inhalation in the air passage. Atypical drowning is often referred to as dry drowning. Water enters the nasopharynx and larynx, causing severe laryngeal spasms and eventual closure. In dogs, aspirating 5 mL of salt or fresh water can result in rapid and persistent hypoxia without producing

Aspiration of 5 mL of salt or fresh water in dogs can cause immediate and persistent hypoxia without producing severe hypercarbia.

Mode of death in drowning

The reasons of death in drowning include asphyxia, shock, and lethal injuries. Asphyxia is the most common cause. Death occurs after five minutes of total submergence.

Clinical findings

Symptoms in affected animals include tachypnea, dyspnea, and tachycardia. Mucous membrane congestion and cyanosis. During lung auscultation, there is a decrease in the usual air flow and noises, which can occur in any location of auscultation. Consolidation of the lung can be detected using thoracic radiography. Hypoxia and metabolic acidosis are present.

Necropsy findings suggestive of death by drowning

The typical indicators of drowning are only obvious if the body is removed from the water and inspected within a few hours following death. Depending on how long the body has been putrefied, these symptoms may change over time or disappear totally when the carcass is recovered from putrification. If there are no evidence of drowning, the corpse should be thoroughly inspected for alternative causes of death such as poisoning, violence, or disease.

Rigor mortis occurs rapidly as a result of muscle effort. Skin seems to be corrugated. If the animal was still alive when it drowned, its injuries would cause an inflammatory reaction. The eyes are either half-open or closed, with congested conjunctivae and dilated pupils. Fine foam from the mouth and nostrils is a telltale sign of drowning.

When the thorax is opened, the lungs expand out of the thoracic cavity because they are spongy, edematous, and balloon-like due to the presence of water. Blood-stained frothy fluid flows away from the sliced surfaces of the lungs during sectioning. The respiratory passages (larynx, trachea, and bronchial tubes) contain fine froth that is periodically stained with blood and foreign material such as sand, mud, algae, and weeds. There could be feed particles that have been regurgitated. The right side of the heart and major veins become dilated as a result of pulmonary circulation blockage. A large volume of water in the stomach and intestine including material such as sand, dirt, and algae from the time of immersion.

Diagnosis

The diagnosis of drowning is complicated. For the diagnosis, an accurate history of drowning and a reliable witness at the site are sufficient. The degree of respiratory compromise is determined through a physical examination, pulse oximetry, and arterial blood gas analysis. Clinical observations and necropsy lesions in dead animals can provide additional support.

Treatment

If a patient drowns, they require immediate emergency care. The points indicated below should be followed.

- Remove the patient from the water immediately.
- Position the patient on their side, extending their head and neck.
- To prevent aspirating stomach contents and promote water drainage from the lungs, keep the head slightly lower than the body.
- Gently push the chest and stomach walls to expel water from the lungs and stomach. Pull the tongue forward; be careful not to get bitten by dogs or cats.
- Provide CPR if necessary.
- To avoid further heat loss, wrap a blanket around the animal.

Treatment for respiratory distress induced by many types of pulmonary sickness is similar to that for drowning. Any patient suffering from respiratory problems requires oxygen therapy, which should be administered quickly. Treatment for hypothermia, shock, and other comorbidities should also be provided. Drowning victims may have consumed large amounts of water, resulting in electrolyte imbalances and putting them in danger of emesis with aspiration. So, if the patient's respiration is stable, nasogastric intubation should be used to drain the stomach of water.

Animals saved from drowning are treated with nasal insufflations of humidified oxygen and sodium bicarbonate, as well as lactated Ringer's solution to rectify the base deficiency. Bronchodilators and nonsteroidal anti-inflammatory drugs can also be employed. Following an antibiotic sensitivity test, antibacterials are given to keep microbes from entering the lungs during drowning.

Key points for management of drowning patients	
1.	Provide oxygen therapy
2.	Dry animal thoroughly and provide warmth to treat hypothermia
3.	Hypovolemia should be treated with appropriate fluid resuscitation
4.	If the stomach contains fluid, consider placing nasogastric tube to remove gastric contents
5.	Provide supportive care- Fluid therapy, bronchodilators, non-steroidal anti-inflammatory drugs
6.	Monitor vital signs and Complete Blood Count, thoracic radiography for evidence of pneumonia

References

Beausoleil N, Mellor D. Introducing breathlessness as a significant animal welfare issue. N Z Vet J. 2015;63(1):44–51.

Beynon J. "Not waving, not drowning." Asphyxia and torture: the myth of simulated drowning and other forms of torture. Torture. 2012;22(S1):25–29.

Bhardwaj W, Mohan M, Rai UC. Electrocardiographic changes in experimental drowning. Indian J Physiol Pharmacol. 1982;26(1):85–89.

Boer J de, Biewenga TJ, Kuipers HA, den Otter G. The effects of aspirated and swallowed water in drowning: sea-water and fresh-water experiments on rats and dogs. Anesthesiology. 1970;32(1):51–59.

Conn AW, Miyasaka K, Katayama M, Fujita M, Orima H, Barker G, Bohn D. A canine study of cold water drowning in fresh versus salt water. Crit Care Med. 1995; 23(12):2029-37.

Karch SB. Pathology of the lung in near-drowning. Am J Emerg Med. 1986;4(1):4–9.

Lunetta P, Modell JH, Sajantila A. What is the incidence and significance of "dry-lungs" in bodies found in water? Am J Forensic Med Pathol. 2004;25(4):291–301.

Lunetta P, Modell JH. Macroscopical, microscopical, and laboratory findings in drowning victims: a comprehensive review. In: Tsokos M, ed. Forensic Pathology Reviews. Totowa, NJ: Humana Press; 2005:3–77.

McEwen BJ, Gerdin J. Veterinary Forensic Pathology: Drowning and bodies recovered from water. Veterinary Pathology. 2016;53(5):1049-1056.

Modell JH, Gaub M, Moya F, Vestal B, Swarz H. Physiological effect of near drowning with chlorinated fresh water, distilled water and isotonic saline. Anesthesiology. 1966;27:33–41.

Modell JH, Moya F, Newby EJ, Ruiz BC, Showers A V. The effects of fluid volume in seawater drowning. Ann Intern Med. 1967;67:68–80.

12

Constipation

Kumari Chandrakala

Key Points

- Constipation can be caused by a variety of clinical disorders or as a subsequent consequence.
- Rehydration and gentle lubrication of the GIT tract with oral paraffin or linseed oil will alleviate constipation caused by feed and water.
- Small animals, especially cats, are more prone to constipation.
- Common treatments for constipation include dietary changes, enemas, and mechanical removal under anesthesia.

Introduction

Constipation occurs when the ingesta moves slowly or not at all. It is a sign of several intestinal disorders. Although not all extra-gastrointestinal illnesses cause constipation, some do. A systemic illness is characterized by parasympathetic nervous system depression and constipation. Many diseases can lead to constipation as a complication. Chronic constipation in dogs leads to obstipation, which is characterized by drier, firmer, and more compact stools. Dogs cannot defecate and hence require medical intervention, such as surgery or manual feces evacuation. When the colon becomes irreversibly swollen and hypomotile (megacolon), surgery may be necessary. As a result, corrective actions for constipation should be implemented as soon as they are discovered. This will aid in a quick recovery from disease. The current chapter provides an overview of constipation in general and its management.

Symptoms

- Excessive straining during defecation.
- Hard, dry faces with pebble-like consistency.
- Repeated straining to defecate can indicate constipation. The most common outcome is defecation failure.
- Some animals may exhibit cracks or fissures in their anal sphincters.

- Cracks or fissures in the anal region might cause fresh blood to appear on feces.
- Signs and symptoms include belly pain, discomfort, loss of appetite, weakness, sunken eyes, a rough body coat, lethargy, and bloating.
- Examining the rectum reveals an engorged hard mass with mucus.
- In severe conditions, dogs and cats may vomit as well.

Etiology

The most common circumstances where constipation has been observed are as follows:

- Common gastrointestinal disorders include diminished peristaltic movement, large intestine impaction, expanded colon, hepatic disorder, peritonitis, anal gland disorder, enlarged prostate, malignancies, and spinal damage.
- Systemic disorders include hypothyroidism and kidney disease.
- Food and habit-related factors include lack of a fibrous diet, dehydration, excessive consumption of finely ground grains or flour, leftovers from festivals or weddings, blockages from non-food items (garbage, bones, placenta, gravel, or plant), and excessive self-grooming, which can cause hair to collect in the stool.
- Common management issues include unexpected dietary changes, stress, anxiety, medication, surgery, and anesthesia.
- Physiological: end stage of pregnancy.
- Older age.

Constipation is a common issue for domestic cats. Intraluminal blockage caused by a variety of triggering factors (mostly dietary or habit-related) is more common. In senior cats, poor digestibility, ingestion of hair (extreme self-grooming), bone, or litter (if confined), and other factors might lead to constipation. Extra-luminal causes, such as compression of the rectum or colon, can cause constipation. Cats can have constipation due to very rare intrinsic (i.e., neuro-muscular dysfunction) reasons.

The clinical conditions indicated above may be explored further to determine their underlying etiology. Pregnancy in the advanced stage causes the gastrointestinal (GIT) movement to slow down in order to keep the fetus alive until full term. This has frequently been observed in high-yielding animals. As a result, it must be handled by providing an appetizing soft feed, plenty of water, and minimizing stress at this time.

Treatment

Large animals

- The first step in managing constipation is injecting NSS or DNS at 5%.
- For non-complicated constipation, liquid paraffin (3-5 L per adult calf) or linseed oil (500-800 mL) can be administered orally alongside NSS or DNS.
- Use 500-1000 g magnesium sulfate per cattle (avoid if there is a blockage, leakage, or perforation of the GIT).
- Cattle and calves can be administered 250-500 g of BOVILAX® or Lax-O-Lax® (bovine luxative) orally with water on a daily basis.
- Higher doses of dewarmer may be beneficial for non-pregnant cattle or calves.
- Surgery is the last resort in life-threatening situations.

Cat and dogs

- Enema

Administration may correct the mild to moderate constipation. In rare cases, manual evacuation of faces is required.

Enema includes

- Warm tap water at 5–10 mL/kg body weight.
- Warm isotonic saline at 5–10 mL/kg BW.
- Dioctyl sodium sulfosuccinate at 5–10 mL per cat.
- Mineral oil at 5–10 mL per cat.
- Lactulose at 5–10 mL per cat.

Note: Tap water or isotonic saline can be used alone or with soap; it is an irritant; others are mild, smooth the lumen, and should be administered using a 10-12-inch French catheter (made of rubber). Enemas containing phosphate should be avoided in cats.

- Rectal suppositories

Constipation is more common in pediatric patients and can be addressed with rectal suppositories. It contains either dioctyl sodium sulfosuccinate (an emollient laxative), glycerin (a lubricating laxative), or bisacodyl. Rectal suppositories can help patients with minor constipation. Oral laxatives, combined with rectal suppositories, are more effective.

- Emollient laxatives

Emollient laxatives such as disoctyl sodium sulfosuccinate and disoctyl calcium sulfosuccinate are administered orally or via enema.

- Docusate sodium: 50 mg capsule per day for cats, 1-4 capsules for dogs based on weight.
- Docusate calcium: 50 mg capsule (1-2 capsules) per day for cats, 2-3 capsules for dogs.

- Dietary fibre

It is well tolerated and preferred because of its effectiveness and physiological tolerability compared to laxatives.

- Psyllium at 1–4 tsp/meal
- Wheat bran at 1–2 tsp/meal
- Pumpkin at 1–4 tsp/meal

The dietary fiber listed above is advised as a complement to canned foods. Animals should be kept hydrated; otherwise, there is a risk of impaction (which is common in the colon).

- Try taking ranitidine and nizatidine at the usual dose.
- Dogs can benefit from probiotics, pumpkin puree, olive oil, apple cider vinegar, and coconut oil.

Note: The treatment enlisted above must be supplemented with the specific treatment of the underlying cause of constipation.

Supportive measures

- Mild activity
- Vitamin B-Complex

Delicious fibrous feed or fodder with plenty of water.

References

ByAlice Defarges , DVM, DACVIM, Department of Clinical Studies, Ontario Veterinary College, University of Guelph Reviewed/Revised Jun 2020 | Modified Oct 2022

CINVEX- Current Indian Veterinary Index PDF,July 12, 2020 by sajeedvet.

Handbook of Veterinary Practitioners Unknown Binding - 1 January 2008 by Dash S.K. (Author)

https://rufusandcoco.com.au/blogs/blog/how-to-make-a-dog-poop-quickly-must-read-guide.

https://www.webmd.com/pets/dogs/dog-constipation-causes-treatment.

13

Diarrhoea

Safeeda Sultana Begum

Key Points

- Neonatal diarrhea can be lethal without treatment.
- Administer aggressive fluid and electrolyte therapy to address newborn diarrhea.
- Fecal examination and/or culture findings can help control diarrhea.
- Ringer lactate is the preferred fluid.
- There is a high association between animal age and the presence of the causal factor for diarrhea.

Introduction

Diarrhea is one of the symptoms of a variety of medical problems. Diarrhea is characterized by an increased frequency of defecation and stools of varied consistency, which may have an increased concentration of water or a decrease in dry matter content. Increased peristaltic movement causes an increase in caudal flow of ingesta/GIT content, resulting in a decrease in intestinal transit time and thus diarrhea. Diarrhea is lethal in children; therefore, preventing fluid and electrolyte losses prior to diagnosis is critical to saving lives.

Etiology

Diarrhea can have a variety of causes. Most of the time, the causal agent is present inside the body. Young neonates are most typically infected by the causal agent found in the dam's feces. Bacterial and viral agents created severe diarrhea, whereas GI parasites caused mild diarrhea. According to the intensity and frequency of recurrence, etiologies are summarized as follows:.

1. Infectious pathogens can disrupt the normal function of gastrointestinal receptors, leading to diarrhea.

Examples: Virus: Rotavirus, Bovine Viral Diarrhea virus, Transmissible Gastroenteritis virus, Parvovirus, Corona virus, and more. Bacteria include *E. coli*, *Salmonella* spp., *Clostridium* spp., *Campylobacter* spp., Gastrointestinal parasites: *Ascaris*, *Trichuris*, *Ancylostoma*, *Strongylus*, and others. Protozoa: *Isospora*, *Eimeria*, Coccidia, *Giardia,* etc. Fungi include *Candid* spp. and *Aspergillus* sp., among others.

Virus and bacterial diarrhea are more common in young animals, but GI parasite-induced diarrhea is clinically recognized in adults. The complications of newborn diarrhea are severe and can be deadly.

2. Chemical agents include arsenic, lead, cobalt, selenium, copper shortage, and toxicity.
3. Poisonous plants include Tulp, Slangkop, and grains with mold infection.
4. Poisoning with organophosphate chemicals.
5. Drug-induced: tetracycline, henylbutazone, etc.
6. Nutritional issues may include acidosis from grain overload, excessive green feed, dietary allergies, and more.
7. Secondary complications of diarrhea include liver disease, peritonitis (hardware disease), heart failure, and chemical or plant poisonings (e.g., lead or nitrate).
8. Miscellaneous causes include metabolic disorders and malignancies.

Clinical findings

- Affected animals exhibit depression, dehydration, emaciation, and malnutrition because they feces with high water loss.
- Protein-losing enteropathy can cause oedema and ascites, while anorexia, nutrient steatorrheoa, and protein-losing enteropathy can cause weight loss.
- Large bowel involvement can lead to frequent defecation, urgency of the tenesmus, and the presence of red blood.
- Small bowel involvement can cause symptoms such as steatorrhea, weight loss, emaciation, and flatulence, while big bowel involvement is less likely to cause these symptoms.

Management

- Start fluid and electrolyte therapy immediately, regardless of clinical indications of dehydration. Oral electrolyte solutions may be useful in the early stages.
- Calves that are recumbent, have a water loss of $\geq 8\%$ of their body weight, or are unable to consume fluids orally require intravenous therapy. These calves are typically acidotic, and the fluid and base deficits can be corrected initially by rapidly administering a hypertonic solution of

sodium bicarbonate (either 500 mL of a 4.2% solution or 250 mL of an 8.4% solution), followed by a physiologically balanced electrolyte solution administered at up to 40 mL/kg/hour until the volume deficit is corrected. Because diarrheal calves are typically hypoglycemic, adding 25-50 g of dextrose to the IV fluids can be useful in the early stages of treatment.

- Parenteral antibiotic therapy should be explored when calves are systemically ill, but diarrhea alone does not warrant treatment. Field investigations demonstrated that at least 30% of diarrheal calves with systemic illness are bacteremic, indicating a strong need for parenteral antibiotic therapy. Because E. coli causes the majority of bacteremia and septicemia in neonatal calves, the chosen antibiotic should be effective against gram-negative bacteria.
- Combining NSAIDs with fluid therapy resulted in speedier recovery, less discomfort, and improved weight gain during the reconvalescent period. The first step in extreme conditions is to keep the body's fluid and electrolyte levels stable. Ringer lactate is the initial choice, and it is administered aggressively to sustain fluid loss within 4-6 hours. If the pharyngeal reflex is maintained, oral rehydration therapy should be administered with caution in patients.
- KCl is suggested for hypokalemia. Meanwhile, a fecal examination for gastrointestinal parasites or culture may enhance the medication.
- Anti-diarrheal medicines and antibiotics should be administered based on the patient's condition, including the suspected or proven origin and composition of the fecal material.
- Astringent and anti-motility medications should be provided as needed.
- To treat parasitic diarrhea, use suitable anthelmintics. Animal feces are examined at regular intervals, and a dewormer is selected accordingly.
- Manage diarrhea caused by chemical agents (Arsenic, Lead), cobalt or selenium deficiency, copper deficiency or toxicity, poisonous plants (Tulp, Slangkop), cereals with mold contamination, nitrate poisoning, and organophosphate poisoning. Tetracycline, phenylbutazone, and other drugs can cause nutrition problems (acidosis, lush green feed, overfeeding, food allergy, etc.) Diarrhea as a secondary result (liver disease, peritonitis, heart failure, etc.) and other causes (metabolic illnesses, malignancies, etc.) are treated by correcting the specific cause, which varies depending on the etiology.

References

A text book of the diseases of cattle, sheep, pigs, goats and horses by Radostits O. M., Gay C. C., Blood D. C. and Hinchcliff K.W., 10th edition, Saunders Publication.

Diarrhea in Neonatal Ruminants by Walter Grünberg in MSD Veterinary manual, Reviewed/ Revised Feb 2021. https: // www.msdvetmanual.com/digestive-system/intestinal-diseases-in-ruminants/diarrhea-in-neonatal-ruminants

14

Dehydration

Anand Mohan

Key Points

- Fluid therapy is crucial for saving dehydrated animals.
- Fluid therapy should be administered within the first 4-6 hours of treatment.
- Ringer lactate is the recommended fluid for diarrhea and enteritis.
- Fluid loss of 4–6 % does not require therapy and does not show any clinical indications.

Introduction

Dehydration is defined as an excessive loss of water and electrolytes from the body (usually due to vomiting and/or diarrhea) or an insufficient intake of water. The body loses water through respiration; however, the skin, face, and/or urine can also cause dehydration. Diarrhea (the loss of fluid and electrolytes from the gastrointestinal tract) is invariably accompanied by dehydration. Chapter 13 provides a brief overview of diarrhea and how it is managed. Dehydration causes lethargy in the patient and, if handled, can have catastrophic consequences for the kidneys and/or other internal organs. Death may occur if the body loses 40% of its water.

Causes of dehydration

Dehydration is a clinical symptom seen in a wide range of illnesses. Dehydration can be caused by a variety of factors.

1. Inadequate water intake
2. Excessive fluid loss is most often associated with infectious agents.

Clinical manifestation

Common indications of dehydration include sunken eyes, loss of subcutaneous suppleness, muscular weakness, inappetence or anorexia, oliguria, and so on. Weight loss can also occur quickly during dehydration. Physical examination of animals using the following methods may aid in the determination of the degree of dehydration.

1. Dehydration causes dryness in the gums and tongue. Saliva gets thick and ropey. Sunken or dried eyes.
2. Skin tent test: Tent the upper eyelid or neck skin; if it takes longer to return to its original position, it may indicate moderate to severe dehydration (Table 14.1).
3. Packed cell volume and total protein: Increased packed cell volume and total serum protein content in serum or plasma indicate dehydration. Fluid deficit is computed, and fluid therapy is recommended (see Tables 14.1 and 14.2).

Table 14.1. Assessment of dehydration on the basis of skin tent test

Skin fold persist (Second)	PCV (%)	% Loss	Fluid required (ml/kg body weight) to replace deficit
-	40-45	4-6	20-25
2-4	50	6-8	30-50
6-10	55	8-10	50-80
20-45	60	10-12	80-120
Prolonged	>60	12-15	>120

Table 14.2. Packed cell volume and severity of fluid therapy

Packed cell volume	Indication
30-40%	Normal
40-50 %	Fluid therapy may or may not be necessary
50% -60%	Fluids are necessary for recovery
> 60%	Intensive fluid therapy is necessary and the prognosis is unfavourable

Management of dehydration

The fluid deficit needs to be maintained as soon as possible. Dehydration can sometimes result in electrolyte losses as well. In this case, each electrolyte's measurement may be necessary, and fluids are picked accordingly. Fluid will be replaced in all conditions of dehydration using the methods listed below.

1. For replacement or hydration therapy, it is recommended to provide it within the first 4-6 hours. The determined fluid volume will be administered by the intravenous route. It will increase circulating blood volume while stabilizing the heart and circulatory system. As a result, essential organs will continue to receive appropriate perfusion. It also assists in maintaining an electrolyte imbalance.
2. Maintenance therapy addresses the daily fluid loss caused by regular animal activity. Feed and water intake are limited or missing in illness patients. However, fluid loss in normal physiology continues; therefore,

maintenance therapy is required until the animal's normal feed and water intake are restored. The amount is computed for 24-hour losses and will be distributed over a 24-hour period. It will sustain recovered blood volume and aid in the early recovery from alignment. It is best administered by intravenous route. The oral route is sometimes recommended if the animal's feed and water intake are normal, and the GIT system is functioning properly. Each medical state has a particular fluid demand. The electrolytes that are depleted differ.

As a result, the selection and quantity of fluid are critical for disease treatment. Table 14.3 lists some of the illnesses conditions and the necessary fluids. In some cases, incorrect fluid therapy can be harmful; Table 14.4 lists some of the diseases for which fluids are contraindicated. If an electrolyte evaluation facility is available, it may augment fluid therapy, as electrolyte supplementation is suggested in fluid. Table 14.5 lists some of the most frequent fluids with electrolyte concentrations. They are classified into several categories based on their osmolarity. Fluids are selected based on the type of dehydration present in each clinical condition.

Table 14.3. Choicc in some disease conditions

Vomiting/gastritis	**Normal Saline Solution (NSS)**
Obstructive urolithiasis	NSS
Diarrhoea/enteritis	Ringer lactate (RL)
Gastrointestinal stasis	RL

Table 14.4. Contraindications of fluid in some disease condition

Fluid	**Contraindication**
5 % Dextrose (D5)	Milk fever, blood transfusion
Dextrose Normal Saline (DNS) / NSS	Ascites, edema
RL	Milk fever
RL	Liver dysfunction, rumen acidosis, metabolic alkalosis, congestive heart failure

Table 14.5. Different type of fluids

Types of solutions	**Isotonic**	**Hypotonic**	**Hypertonic**	**Colloids**
Examples	• 0.9% Sodium chloride (NSS)	• 0.45% Sodium Chloride	• 3% Sodium Chloride	• Haemecal
	• DNS (0.9 NaCl and 5% dextrose)	• 0.33% Sodium Chloride	• D20, D25, Sodium Bicarbonate 5%	• 20% Mannitol
	• Lactated Ringer's solution		• Protein solutions	• Dextran

Calculation of fluid deficit:

Volume of fluid in liter = body weight (in kg) x % of dehydration

Note

1. Dehydration percentage can be estimated using the skin tent test (Table 14.1), packed cell volume (Table 14.1, 14.2), or electrolyte concentration in serum or plasma.
2. The usual daily maintenance dose is 50 mL per kg body weight of the animal.
3. The most common way to administer fluids is intravenously, which can deliver a substantial amount of fluid. Intravenous delivery is favored for hypertonic and isotonic fluids. Further high volumes will be provided in a short period of time; therefore, hydration therapy will be administered completely via the intravenous route. Oral route - suggested if water or food consumption and GIT function are normal. As a result, this approach may be used for maintenance therapy in the recovery stage of animals. Subcutaneously, only isotonic solutions can be administered. Intra-peritoneal is desirable in hypothermic new born.

References

Jadhav, Y.B., Bhojne G.R., Dakshinkar N.P., Kurkure N.V. and Rangnekar M.N. (2020). Oral rehydration of adult cattle using isotonic solution of sugar, sodium chloride and potassium chloride. Haryana Vet. 59(SI): 93-95.

Textbook of Veterinary Medicine. Sharma, MC., Mahesh Kumar and Sharma, R.D. (Ed.), ICAR, Krishi Anusandhan Bhavan, Pusa, New Delhi.

UBC ACC Guidelines and SOP for the Maintenance of Fluid Homeostasis in Animals, 2018. Available at https://animalcare.ubc.ca/sites/default/files/documents/Maintenance%20of%20Fluid%20Homeostasis%20Dec%202018.pdf

Veterinary Medicine: A textbook of the diseases of cattle, horses, sheep, pigs and goat. O. M. Radostits C.C.Gay, K.W. Hinchcliff, P.D. Constable (Ed.), 10th edition. Saunders, Elsevier.

15

Vomiting

Neelam Kushwaha

Key Points

- Vomiting is a common sign of various conditions, including irritants and toxins, kidney or liver failure, pancreatitis, neurological disorders, and digestive issues. Common in dogs and cats.
- Can be fatal in horses with acute stomach dilatation.
- Ruminants (cattle, buffalo, sheep, and goats) vomit by regurgitating ruminal material through their mouths.

Introduction

Vomiting is the violent ejection of stomach and, on occasion, proximal small intestine contents through the mouth caused by fierce contractions of the diaphragm and abdominal muscles. It is the most prevalent protective disruption in the gastrointestinal system. Vomiting has three distinct phases: nausea, retching, and vomiting. A sense of nausea may or may not cause vomiting. Nausea is scientifically defined as sadness, salivation, lip-licking, and increased swallowing motions in animals. Retching is caused by a series of spasmodic respiratory movements involving the closed glottis. Vomiting is characterized by repeated thoracic invaginations of the abdominal esophagus and cardia. Projectile vomiting often occurs when an animal begins to vomit without going through three stages.

Vomiting is typical in both dogs and cats. It is a deadly sign in horses that occurs with acute gastric dilation. In agricultural animals, vomiting has a very dismal prognosis. In ruminants (cattle, buffalo, sheep, and goats), vomiting is the regurgitation of a large volume of ruminal content through the mouth. Regurgitation must be distinguished from vomiting. It is the release of food from the esophagus or stomach without the contraction of abdominal muscles. Regurgitation usually happens right after you eat or drink something. When cattle regurgitate, the ejected food and liquid are often undigested and may resemble the cylindrical shape of an oesophagus. Regurgitation is usually followed by coughing or trouble breathing rather than vomiting.

Etiology

Vomiting can be caused by a variety of diseases in diverse animal species. Vomiting is common following the ingestion of irritants and poisons, renal or liver failure, pancreatitis, neurological system disorders, digestive system diseases, and so on.

Dogs and cats

- Drug-induced: aspirin and phenylbutazone.
- Conditions include hepatitis, nephritis, pyometra, and pancreatitis.
- Metabolic diseases include diabetes and hyperthyroidism.
- Lead and zinc poisoning.
- Gastritis, acute gastroenteritis, stomach dilatation, ulcers, and hypomotility.
- Common food-related issues include food poisoning, allergies, intolerances, and consuming stale or decomposed food.
- Foreign body in -esophagus or stomach.
- A hiatus hernia.
- Parasitic infection.

Cattle, buffalo, sheep and goat (regurgitation)

- Cud dropping due to faulty molar teeth
- Arsenic poisoning
- Plant poisoning (Oleander spp. or Kaner)
- Fluid overdose in the rumen
- Pharyngeal paralysis or paresis

Pig

- Vomiting and wasting illness.
- Infection with the Haemagglutinating Encephalomyelitis Virus.
- Acute chemical poisoning.
- Fungal poisoning.

Clinical findings

- Vomiting may be continuous, intermittent, or projectile-type.
- Vomitus can vary in substance, odor, and color depending on its origin.
- In chronic gastritis, stomach ulcers, drug-induced erosion, and neoplasia, vomiting may contain new blood (haematemesis).

- Vomiting with a fecal odor may indicate intestinal blockage, peritonitis, or ischaemia.
- Aspiration pneumonia is a dangerous complication of vomiting.

Diagnosis

The presence of a concurrent disease condition, a history of consuming strange foods, a history of poisoning, clinical indicators, the beginning and frequency of vomiting, and the intensity of the symptoms (mild, moderate, or severe) all aid in diagnosis.

It is critical to get a blood test, and particular biochemical testing for the liver, kidneys, and pancreas. Contrast radiography, ultrasonography, and endoscopy are recommended for the diagnosis of numerous gastrointestinal illnesses associated with vomiting.

Treatment

Vomiting is a typical clinical sign of numerous illnesses. The treatment differs depending on the exact cause. The primary goals of treatment are to remove the irritant, control vomiting, and correct fluid, electrolyte, and acid-base imbalances. Monitoring patients is critical. It is recommended to check the patient's vital signs every 4-8 hours, as well as the PCV, glucose, BUN, and electrolyte levels every 8-24 hours.Nothing should be given orally until the patient's vomiting has been controlled. As a result, it is recommended that you fast for 24-48 hours. If the vomiting has stopped after 24 hours, provide a modest amount (approximately a teaspoonful) of bland, readily digestible food. If there are no further instances of vomiting, feeding can usually be gradually resumed.Ice cubes can be fed to lick to quench thirst and do not cause vomiting.

Vomiting causes Na, K, and Cl losses; thus, normal saline solution (0.9%) is the preferred fluid for treating metabolic alkalosis. The type and amount of fluid to be administered are determined by the frequency and severity of vomiting. Fluid treatment is required to correct dehydration and electrolyte abnormalities over a period of 2-6 hours (for critically ill patients) or 8-12 hours.

Along with this, vomiting is treated with the use of the following drugs:

i. H2 receptor antagonists or antacid-
    - *Ranitidine @2 mg/kg body weight PO or IV or IM q8-12h*
    - *Cimetidine @5-10 mg/kg body weight PO q8h*
    - *Famotidine @ 0.5–1 mg/kg body weight IV or PO Q 12–24 h*

ii. Proton pump inhibitors
   - *Omeprazole @0.7 mg/kg body weight PO q 24 h*
   - *Pantoprazole @ 0.7–1 mg/kgbody weight PO or IV q 24 h*

iii. Antiemetics
   - *Metoclopramide @ 0.2-0.5 mg/kg body weight PO q 8 h*
   - *Ondansetron @ 0.5-1 mg/kgbody weight IV q 24 horq12-24 h*
   - *Phenothiazine tranquilizer e.g.Chlorpromazine @ 0.2-0.4 mg/kgbody weight SC or IM q 8 h.*

   (Phenothiazine tranquilizer must be used with great caution in the case of dehydration).

iv. Cytoprotective agent-for treating gastro-intestinal ulcers.

   Sucralfate @ 0.25–1 g PO q 8–12 h.

References

MSD Veterinary manual. Available at https://www.msdvetmanual.com/dog-owners/digestive-disorders-of-dogs/vomiting-in-dogs

Textbook of Clinical Veterinary Medicine by MC Sharma, Mahesh Kumar and RD Sharma(2009). Directorate of Information and Publications of Agriculture, ICAR. PP: 78-80.

16

Seizures

Neelam Kushwaha

Key Points

- Seizures are common in dogs and cats but uncommon in larger animals.
- Animal seizures can be induced by several circumstances.
- Idiopathic epilepsy is the leading cause of seizures.
- Rapidly rising core body temperature and metabolic alterations lead to fatal outcomes.

Introduction

A seizure is defined as any rapid and uncontrollable movement of the body induced by aberrant neuronal activity in the brain. Seizures are common in dogs and cats, but uncommon in larger animals. Seizures can be severe, affecting the entire body, or moderate, affecting only a section of the body. The pet may or may not be conscious or responsive, and it may urinate.

Seizures are usually brief (1-2 minutes) and self-limiting; however, some animals may experience protracted activity (more than 5 minutes). Seizures that persist longer than 3 to 5 minutes might cause serious complications such as pulmonary or brain edema. Death is caused by a sudden rise in body temperature and metabolic alterations that reach a life-threatening threshold.

Etiology

Seizures are prevalent in dogs and cats. Epilepsy, otitis media, toxins, hypoglycemia, brain tumors, metabolic disturbances (diabetes mellitus, uraemia, hepatic coma, alkalosis, hypocalcaemia), cardiac diseases (aortic stenosis, pulmonary stenosis, myocardial infarction, etc.), distemper, roundworm and tapeworm infestations, and a variety of other medical conditions can all cause it.

Reactive seizures occur as a result of metabolic abnormalities such as hypoglycemia, hypercalcemia, liver disease, hepatic shunts, and renal illness. In this situation, the brain is normal. The seizures go away if the metabolic issue is managed.

Toxic substances may potentially cause seizures. This is a risk associated with goods like dark chocolate, caffeine, xylitol, and rat poison. Seizures are resolved by removing the toxin and administering medication to correct the toxicity.

Seizures can be caused by brain abnormalities such as tumors, trauma, inflammatory illnesses, and infectious diseases including rabies and canine distemper. This is known as a structural seizure.

Idiopathic epilepsy is the leading cause of seizures. Idiopathic epilepsy is a disorder of unknown origin that is often diagnosed after all other possible causes have been eliminated. Idiopathic epilepsy often develops between the ages of six months and six years. A breed propensity to epilepsy is another factor that can help with diagnosis. Schnauzers, Collies, Bassett Hounds, Cocker Spaniels, Labrador Retrievers, and Golden Retrievers are more likely than other breeds to have seizure problems.

Seizures in animals under one year of age are typically caused by a birth abnormality, such as hydrocephalus or a portosystemic shunt.

Symptoms

Seizures are usually characterized by loss of consciousness, uncontrollable convulsions, salivation, urine, and an elevated heart rate. However, some animals with seizures do not exhibit all of the standard clinical indications, making diagnosis problematic.

Status epilepticus is a condition in which seizures occur continuously, one after the other, without interruption. This can lead to an irreversible coma or death; thus, it should be addressed as a medical emergency.

Treatment

There are several reasons that might trigger seizures in animals. While it is vital to lessen the frequency of seizures, disregarding possible underlying causes is not recommended.

- Identify the etiology of epilepsy by conducting a complete history, physical examination, laboratory examination, radiography, MRI, spinal fluid analysis, EEG, and cerebral angiography before starting treatment.
- To prevent self-inflicted trauma or mishaps, keep the animal in a safe environment.
- To treat status epilepticus, create an airway and provide oxygen.
- If the temperature remains high, an ice bath can be administered.
- If cerebral edema is detected, oxygen, mannitol, or corticosteroids may be given.When there is no clear extracranial source of the seizure

disease, anticonvulsant medication can be initiated. A wide range of medications can be used to treat seizures.

Dogs and cats

Diazepam is the most often used treatment for seizures in dogs and cats. When given intravenously (0.5-2 mg/kg), the dose may be repeated up to three times at 5- to 10-minute intervals. If seizures occur after the second or third intravenous dose, a diazepam continuous-rate infusion (CRI) at 0.5-2 mg/kg/hr may be more beneficial. When used as a CRI, diazepam should be combined with either 5% dextrose or 0.9% saline. It should not be used with lactated Ringer's solution, as the calcium may precipitate diazepam. Because plastic absorbs diazepam, it should not be kept in plastic syringes or IV settings for long periods of time.

Diazepam has limited usage as a primary anticonvulsant in dogs due to its quick hepatic clearance, short half-life, and rapid development of functional tolerance to the anticonvulsant action. It has, however, been demonstrated to be quite successful in managing seizure disorders when administered orally at 0.5-2.0 mg/kg body weight and repeated every 8 hours. Phenobarbital is commonly used in status epilepticus to prevent more seizure activity. Phenobarbital is the preferred anticonvulsant for cats. Phenobarbital at 3-6 mg/kg, IV or IM, can be given every 15-30 minutes. If injectable phenobarbital is helpful in preventing or managing seizures, an oral maintenance dose may be initiated with the goal of gradually reducing or eliminating injectable anticonvulsant infusions over the following 24 hours.

Note: Both diazepam and phenobarbital should be used with great caution because the potentiation of their effects increases the risk of respiratory and cardiovascular collapse.

Sodium pentobarbital is commonly used to treat uncontrollable seizures in dogs and cats, particularly if diazepam and phenobarbital have failed. To achieve anaesthesia in dogs and cats, it is administered at a dosage of 2-15 mg/kg. Because pentobarbital is a respiratory depressant, respiratory assistance should be easily accessible. When injected perivascularly or subcutaneously, the medication causes irritation. As the animal recovers from the drug's effects, it may experience excitation, which might be misconstrued as seizure activity. If an animal is given phenobarbital, it should undergo a full blood count, serum biochemistry, and liver function tests (bile acids or ammonia).Potassium bromide (KBr) at 22-44 mg/kg PO, administered every 24 hours with meals, can be used to treat seizures in dogs.

Foals and Horses

Diazepam has a prolonged elimination half-life in horses (7-22 hours). The dose for foals is 0.05-0.4 mg/kg, delivered slowly via IV. Higher doses of diazepam in foals can be lethal to the neonates. Diazepam (25-50 mg/horse, IV) can be used to treat seizures in adult horses. To avoid more seizures following the initial diazepam injection, phenobarbital at 12-20 mg/kg IV over 20 minutes may be started as a follow-up and subsequently maintained at a dosage of 6.65-9 mg/kg IV over 20 minutes, b.i.d. or t.i.d. Sedation should be avoided by reducing the dosage.

Ruminants

Diazepam (0.5-1.5 mg/kg, IM or IV) can be used to halt seizures in large ruminants. Pentobarbital (20-30 mg/kg) can be administered intravenously to sheep and goats to induce anaesthesia.

References

Managing seizures. Cornell Richard P. Riney Canine Health Center. Available at: https://www.vet.cornell.edu/departments/riney-canine-health-center/canine-health-information/managing-seizures

MSD Veterinary manual. Aavilable at:https://www.msdvetmanual.com/pharmacology/systemic-pharmacotherapeutics-of-the-nervous-system/anticonvulsants-or-antiepileptic-drugs.

Textbook of Clinical Veterinary Medicine by MC Sharma, Mahesh Kumar and RD Sharma (2009). Directorate of Information and Publications of Agriculture, Indian Council of Agriculture Research.

17

Traumatic Injury

Mamta Mishra

Key Points

- Traumatic injuries occur when an animal injures another or falls or strikes surrounding infrastructure (e.g., flooring, fence, gate).
- Common types of injuries include fractures, dislocations, bruises, and wounds, which might be penetrating or not.

Introduction

Physical injuries may occur throughout the export procedure. Slipping and being trampled or mounted during transportation or yarding are likely the most common causes of severe injuries. Poorly built or maintained facilities, such as yards, laneways, fences, gates, and flooring, can increase the risk of injury to animals while they are kept or handled. Poor stockmanship, such as rough handling and putting too much pressure on others, can also increase the chance of harm. Individual animals can be injured by improper restraint or handling, such as dragging an animal by its front or hind legs.

Types of Traumatic Injuries

- Fractures
- Shock
- Cuts, bruises, and lacerations
- Brain and head injuries
- Internal organ injuries
- Respiratory problem

Clinical signs and diagnosis

An animal that is bright and alert but suddenly loses the ability to stand or move properly is a clear indication of a catastrophic injury. If the animal has died, a necropsy may reveal fractures, dislocations, wounds, subcutaneous bruises, hematoma, cellulitis, or other forms of infection.

Treatment

Animals with wounds should be isolated in a clean environment, and wound management should follow the standard protocol outlined in Chapter: Wound. Lame animals should be taken to a hospital pen with unrestricted trough access. Fractures and dislocated joints necessitate prompt treatment and skill for successful reduction; guidelines for this are briefly discussed in Chapter: Musculoskeletal System. Xylazine sedation or anesthesia may be required to allow decreases.

Traumatic head and brain Injury

Traumatic head injury is common in tiny animals and causes brain impairment. The most prevalent causes are car accidents in dogs and crush injuries in cats.

Treatment

Treatment is primarily concerned with maintaining cerebral circulation, lowering intracranial pressure (ICP), and treating secondary injuries.

Hyperosmolar therapy (mannitol, hypertonic saline) is the preferred treatment for lowering ICP in patients with TBI. Mannitol is recommended as a first-line treatment for TBI patients who are euvolemic and preferably normotensive, according to the Brain Trauma Foundation's human medicine guidelines.

Mannitol is recommended at a dose of 0.5 to 1.5 g/kg administered as a bolus over 15 to 20 minutes. Hypertonic saline may potentially be a preferable option for hypovolemic individuals, although it is contraindicated in hypernatremia. The recommended doses for hypertonic saline are 3 to 4 mL/kg (7.5% sodium chloride [NaCl]) and 5.3 mL/kg (3% NaCl).

When using a peripheral vein, utilize a lower dose of hypertonic saline (3%) because a larger concentration (7.5%) generally induces severe vasculitis. In addition to hyperosmolar treatment, raising the head at a 15° to 30° angle while keeping the head and neck extended reduces cerebral blood volume by improving venous drainage from the brain.

For isotonic crystalloids (e.g., lactated Ringer solution, 0.9% saline), quarter shock doses (based on a shock volume of 90 mL/kg in dogs and 60 mL/kg in cats) administered immediately are recommended (details are provided in chapter: Shock). Synthetic colloids can be administered at a rate of 10 to 20 mL/kg in dogs (maximum 40 mL/kg/h) or 5 mL/kg in cats over 5 to 10 minutes. Fluid therapy should be maintained until appropriate tissue perfusion is achieved (normal heart rate, blood pressure, pulse quality, mucous membrane color, and capillary refill time).

Another alternative for treating hypovolemic or hypotensive shock is hypertonic saline 4 mL/kg (7.5% NaCl) and 5.3 mL/kg (3% NaCl), but its action lasts only 15 to 75 minutes. Hypertonic saline boluses should always be followed by a maintenance dose of isotonic crystalloids. Corticosteroids are not recommended for TBI patients because they have been shown to increase mortality in humans.

Patients' active seizures can be managed with anticonvulsants. The first-line rescue treatment is diazepam or midazolam (0.5 to 1 mg/kg IV or 0.3 to 0.5 mg/kg IV, respectively). After a seizure, a maintenance anticonvulsant drug should be taken to avoid future seizures. Levetiracetam is a solid choice. The loading dose for levetiracetam is 60 mg/kg IV, followed by 30 mg/kg IV every 8 hours. To avoid severe and potentially fatal adverse events, levetiracetam should be diluted as directed on the package insert and delivered slowly over 15 minutes.

Decreased cerebral oxygen delivery is the primary cause of subsequent brain damage. Pulse oximetry is an effective method of evaluating oxygenation status; hence, oxygen supplementation is frequently required.

Adequate pain control is critical for patient comfort and preventing an increase in ICP due to an elevated cerebral metabolic rate. Opioids are widely used. The suggested fentanyl dose is 2-6 μg/kg/hr. Naloxone can be used as a reversal agent if necessary. Patients with TBI have a high metabolic and catabolic rate. Early nutritional support is required to reduce patient mortality. If veterinary patients are unable to eat enough calories, enteral feeding (nasogastric or esophageal tubes) is administered. Metoclopramide (0.2 to 0.5 mg/kg BW) should be taken concurrently, as patients with TBI frequently experience delayed stomach emptying. Antibiotics are recommended in the presence of shock, open wounds, calvarium fractures (particularly basilar or sinus fractures), and foreign material implanted in the brain parenchyma. Antibiotics should be lipid-soluble in order to pass the blood-brain barrier and have antibacterial activities.

Surgical Therapy

In veterinary patients with TBI, craniotomies may be performed to remove epidural or subdural hematomas, decompress skull fractures, remove foreign items embedded in the brain parenchyma, achieve hemostasis, or decompress for gradual neurologic deterioration.

Prevention

Handling facilities should be designed and built to reduce the risk of animal and human injury, and they should be inspected on a regular basis for potential dangers. Personnel should be taught low-stress animal handling to ensure that animals are handled appropriately, reducing stress and injury risk. Animals are classified according to size, gender, and horn length.

At discharge, sick and injured animals should be confined and unloaded separately from healthy animals to avoid trample. Utilize low-stress handling and transportation methods.

Internal organ injuries and respiratory problem

Internal organ damage and open abdominal and respiratory cavities are common in both large and small animals. Symptoms include a quick pulse and shallow breathing, black diarrhea, gum color change (pale or blue), whimpering when touched or moved, glazed eyes, coughing or vomiting blood, bruising or scraping wounds, and a comatose state indicating shock.

Diagnosis of internal injuries

A complete physical examination should be performed unless the animal requires immediate life-saving care. If an animal goes into shock, take quick steps to protect its internal organs. Depending on the animal's condition, diagnostic tests should be recommended [complete blood count (CBC), X-rays, abdominal radiography, electrocardiogram (EKG), and serum chemistry profile]. While fractured bones are evident indicators of trauma, interior damage is critical to evaluate. Bleeding from ruptured organs requires immediate intervention.

Treatment of internal injuries

The treatment will be determined by the underlying cause of the damage. Animals suffering from automobile injuries may need to be hospitalized, particularly at the start of treatment. Oxygen treatment and intravenous fluids may be necessary. Medication for any type of pain will assist, and a professional may recommend antibiotics. If an animal's heart beats wildly as a result of stress or trauma, he may require antiarrhythmic medication. Other therapies may necessitate blood transfusions if animals have lost a significant amount of blood.

Surgery may be required in cases of open cavities, evisceration, sickness (cancer and tumors), fractured bones (particularly spinal or neck bones), and other traumas that animals may sustain. Emergency respiratory problems are treated with appropriate oxygen therapy, either via an endotracheal tube or a temporary or permanent tracheostomy. Chest tube insertion is suggested for removing pulmonary effusions. Intermittent positive pressure breathing must be maintained (as briefly explained in Chapter: Respiratory System).

References

Besenski N (2002). Traumatic injuries: imaging of head injuries. Eur Radiol. 2002;12(6): 1237–1252.

Centers for Disease Control and Prevention. Injury prevention & control: traumatic brain injury & concussion [accessed 2016 Jan 22].

Hardaway RM and Williams CH (1990). A new treatment for traumatic shock and ARDS, Resuscitation, 19(1), 61-76.

Marshall, Lawrence FMD (2000). Head Injury: Recent Past, Present, and Future. Neurosurgery 47(3): 546-561.

18

Shock

Safeeda Sultana Begum

Key Points

- Shock occurs when the circulatory system fails to provide adequate blood flow to essential organs.
- Oxygen deficiency is a clinical condition caused by insufficient oxygen delivery or tissue incapacity to use oxygen effectively.
- Successful shock management requires early recognition, aggressive monitoring, and appropriate interventions.

Introduction

Shock is a complex physiological syndrome marked by widespread circulatory irregularities that result in inadequate tissue perfusion. In other words, it is a clinical condition caused by an insufficient delivery of oxygen to tissues or the tissues' inability to correctly use oxygen. It is a complication of trauma and diseases typically seen in emergency rooms, such as heart failure, inflammatory conditions (e.g., pancreatitis), and sepsis. In shock, tissue perfusion and oxygen delivery are insufficient to support the tissues' baseline metabolic demands. Whatever the cause, shock is distinguished by reduced blood flow, which is typically accompanied by low blood pressure (hypotension).

Shock is defined as anything that causes a severe and typically rapid drop in cardiac output, blood volume, and/or peripheral vascular resistance. Shock is defined as 1) hypovolemic shock, 2) vasogenic shock, 3) endotoxic shock, 4) cardiogenic shock, 5) neurogenic shock, 6) anaphylactic shock, or 7) obstructive shock.

Hypovolemic shock

It is caused by a lack of intravascular circulating blood volume, which is most usually caused by hemorrhage. It can occur as a result of acute blood loss (major lacerations, ruptured thoracic or abdominal organs, surgical procedure) or severe acute fluid loss into the gastrointestinal tract, through the kidneys, or into a "third" space (peritoneal or pleural cavity), severe hemorrhage, and excessive plasma loss caused by burn injury, intestinal obstruction, severe vomiting and diarrhea, diuresis, pancreatitis, and so on. This is the most prevalent type of shock encountered in veterinary patients, characterized by a loss of fluid from the circulating blood volume. It is critical that this type of fluid loss be distinguished from that observed with dehydration.

Vasogenic shock

The body exhibits generalized inappropriate vasodilation, resulting in changes in the pattern of blood flow between tissues. Even with normal blood volume, dilated blood vessels can drastically impair tissue perfusion.

Endotoxic shock or septic shock

This form of shock is mainly caused by poisons produced by bacteria that infiltrate the animals' bodies. Toxin absorption from the colon or mammary glands can also cause endotoxic shock, as demonstrated in cases of acute diffuse peritonitis and coliform mastitis.

Cardiogenic shock

It is induced by insults that reduce cardiac output. This occurs as a result of a variety of cardiac disorders, including advanced (late-stage) cardiomyopathies and valvular disease, as well as severe arrhythmias, myocardial infarction, coronary block, cardiac arrest, acute heart failure, and ventricular fibrillation caused by diminished cardiac output. Anything that alters heart rate or contractility can reduce cardiac output. However, in veterinary medicine, patients with cardiac disease are more likely to exhibit symptoms of congestive heart failure and respiratory difficulties.

Neurogenic shock

Shock can also be caused by pain or depression of the central nervous system. It can happen after severe trauma, intense pain, or, on rare occasions, restraint.

Anaphylactic shock

It is caused by the release of histamine or histamine-like compounds as part of the body's defense response against alien pathogens, which results in an aberrant antigen-antibody reaction. It is the systemic manifestation of an acute hypersensitivity (allergic) reaction.

Obstructive shock

Obstruction of blood flow in big veins. This type of shock is uncommon in veterinary patients, but it can occur with pericardial effusion (when pressure in the pericardial sac restricts venous return to the right side of the heart) or major pulmonary thromboembolism (gastric dilatation and volvulus).

Clinical findings

As the animal's blood volume decreases, several homeostatic mechanisms increase heart rate and stroke volume to maintain cardiac output and tissue perfusion (compensated shock). This causes an irregularity in the pressure parameters (reduction in venous blood pressure), heart rate (increase), pulse (weak), respiration (shallow), and color of the mucous membrane (turns pale from red). Additionally, the animal becomes dull, dejected, feeble, and recumbent. The extremities grow frigid, but the body temperature remains below average. If the condition is not addressed swiftly, the patient will fall into a coma and eventually die.

Diagnosis

The patient's history, as well as clinical symptoms, can assist in the diagnosis of shock. If arterial blood pressure falls below the normal level (typically 120 mm Hg), it may suggest the presence of shock and should be treated right away. Reduced blood pH, as well as a rise in eosinophil count, creatine, and blood urea nitrogen levels, are all signs of shock. ECG (electrocardiography) is useful in identifying cardiogenic shock.

Treatment

The most important goals in the treatment of shock include:

- Diagnose the patient's shock quickly.
- Remove the cause of shock (e.g., hemorrhagic hypovolemia, septic shock).
- Treat the result of shock.
- Supporting crucial functions.
- Ensure patent airways.
- Oxygen treatment.

Hypovolemic shock

Large-volume fluid resuscitation is used to treat hypovolemic shock. Following an assessment of fluid loss, crystalloid solutions (fluids containing electrolytes) or colloid solutions (fluids that increase plasma osmotic pressure and expand plasma volume) can be administered as needed.

- Isotonic RL, 0.9% normal saline, or dextrose solutions can be used at 30-50 ml/kg/hr for big animals, 90 ml/kg/hr for dogs, and 60 ml/kg/hr for cats IV.
- Repeat with colloids such as hetastarch, dextran, and gelatin polymers at a rate of 5-10 ml/kg until the patient stabilizes.

Endotoxic shock

In the event of endotoxic shock, antibiotic treatment in conjunction with fluid therapy is required. A broad-spectrum antibiotic or a combination of antibiotics should be administered for three to five days. Corticosteroids such as dexamethasone at 5- 10 mg/kg body weight are also indicated. The use of cyclooxygenase inhibitors such as flunixin meglumine at 0.2 mg/kg BW is frequently associated with early recovery.

Cardiogenic shock

The treatment is based on the underlying cardiac problem. The primary goal should be to correct the underlying cardiac condition. Fluid treatment is generally not recommended in cardiogenic shock. Positive inotropes (Dobutamine) without fluid treatment may help with myocardial depression.

Obstructive shock

Obstructive shock is primarily concerned with removing the cause for vascular obstruction. For example, performing pericardiocentesis on a patient with pericardial effusion and then administering appropriate treatment based on the underlying reason of vascular obstruction. Gastric dilation and volvulus need surgical intervention.

It is generally difficult to handle vasogenic, neurogenic, and anaphylactic shock. The early detection of the underlying causes of these shocks is quite challenging. However, symptomatic therapy may initially be effective in some cases. Depending on the symptoms, a life-saving medicine may occasionally allow for the diagnosis of the underlying condition.

In addition to all of these treatments, oxygen supplementation, catecholamines, plasma therapy, histamine-2 receptor antagonists (famotidine, ranitidine), and proton pump inhibitors (omeprazole, pantoprazole) to reduce acid production, sucralfate (a gastrointestinal protectant), antiemetics, and so on should be used in conjunction with the primary treatment, depending on the patient's condition.

Reference

A text book of the diseases of cattle, sheep, pigs, goats and horses by Radostits O. M., Gay C. C., Blood D. C. and Hinchcliff K.W., 10th edition, Saunders Publication.

19

Abdominal Pain

Anand Mohan

Key Points

- There are several causes of abdominal pain.
- It is difficult to diagnose in animals, but behavioral changes may indicate abdominal pain.
- Evaluate and treat abdominal pain promptly to avoid life-threatening situations.

Introduction

Abdominal discomfort is typically acute (onset occurs suddenly), although it can also be persistent. It could be caused by inflammation of the abdominal wall or organs in the abdominal and pelvic cavities. Diagnosis is difficult due to the variety of etiologies involved. Patients with stomach pain demonstrate changes in behavior and posture. Treatment should be based on etiology and the underlying cause.

Etiology

Pain can come from the abdominal wall (for example, from trauma), any organ within the abdomen (liver, gallbladder, pancreas, stomach, small intestine, large intestine, adrenal glands, kidneys, bladder, prostate (male animals), ovaries or uterus (female animals), spleen, or abdominal lymph nodes), the lining of the abdomen, or referred pain from another body part (particularly the spine).

Peritonitis, trauma to the abdominal wall, abdominal abscess, hemoperitoneum, pneumoperitoneum, diarrhea, enteritis, gastrointestinal perforation, intestinal obstruction, intussusception, strangulation, volvulus, colic, enterolith, gastric dilatation-volvulus, gastric ulcer, acute pancreatitis, pancreatic abscess/ neoplasia, hepatic abscess, hepatic rupture, chronic hookworm infestation, retained placenta, pyometra, uterine rupture, dystocia, and ovarian cyst.

Clinical signs

Signs vary depending on the underlying cause, but abdominal pain is often characterized by:

- Vocalization, restlessness, and posture changes.
- Difficulty getting out of a lying-down position.
- Pets may bite when picked up or touched under the abdomen.
- Resentment against attempts to touch the abdomen.
- Audible gastrointestinal sounds.
- Obvious abdominal distension or bloating.
- Licking on the flank.
- Dogs with an arched back or "prayer position" may have abdominal pain. This position involves raising the hindquarters and keeping the chest and forelegs close to the ground.
- Tachypnea or tachycardia.
- Colic symptoms in horses include looking back at the flanks, curling the upper lip and arching the neck, continuously elevating a rear leg or kicking the belly, lying down, rolling from side to side, sweating, and stretching out.

Diagnosis

A thorough physical examination of the patient should be conducted. Clinical symptoms, percussion, palpation, and auscultation of the abdomen will aid in determining the cause of pain.

1. ***Abdominal inspection:*** During a distance examination, the contour of the belly provides insight into the diagnosis of abdominal problems. Distension of the abdomen produced by effusion, gastric dilatation, or uroperitoneum is easily identifiable.
2. ***Abdominal palpation:*** This helps to localize pain. A superficial, soft palpation should be conducted. Deep palpation should be done when necessary.
3. ***Percussion and auscultation:*** In dogs with abdominal effusion, percussion detects a fluid wave. Toxin ingestion, acute intestinal blockage, and gastroenteritis all increase the frequency of gut sounds, whereas ileus, anorexia, chronic intestinal obstruction, and abdominal effusions can decrease the frequency of gut sounds.

To determine whether gastrointestinal noises are missing, auscultate the belly and listen for at least 2-3 minutes. In large ruminants, simultaneous percussion and auscultation of the belly to produce a ping sound aid in determining the source of abdominal pain or the damaged organ.

- Rectal palpation can detect caecal dilation and intussusception through dilated intestinal loops, providing valuable diagnostic information.
- A bitch's vulva should be inspected for any discharge (which can be visible in open pyometra).
- Examine the oral cavity for any signs of caustic substance consumption.

Treatment

Treatment for abdominal pain should be determined by the cause and severity of the discomfort. The following therapy should be used to manage stomach pain in general.

Analgesics and anti-inflammatory drugs: It is more necessary to control pain in order to save the animal. Flunixin is a more effective visceral analgesic. Sedatives such as Xylazine HCl (0.2-0.4 mg/kg body weight IV) and butorphanol (0.02-0.1 mg/kg body weight IV) are also utilized for effective pain relief in colic instances.

Fluid treatment is used to hydrate the animal, replenish fluid and electrolyte loss, and enhance circulation. An intravenous infusion of Ringer's lactate is required to maintain electrolyte balance.

Antimicrobial therapy: Broad-spectrum antibiotics must be started when bacterial translocation of the gastrointestinal system is suspected, and they can be given before surgery.

Laxatives and lubricants: Magnesium hydroxide is used to treat intestinal blockage and ileus. Large amounts of NS or DNS (100-150 ml/kg body weight IV) will soften impacted masses in impactive colic.

This book's colic chapter goes into great detail about how to handle colic.

Dogs suffering from abdominal abscess, abdominal wall perforation, gastric dilatation-volvulus, an intestinal foreign body producing pain, intestinal obstruction, or uroperitoneum require immediate treatment. Any delay may end in death.

References

A text book of the diseases of cattle, sheep, pigs, goats and horses by Rodostis O. M., Gay C. C., Blood D. C. and Hinchcliff K.W., 10th edition, Saunders Publication.

KilpatrickS (2015). Abdominal pain and swelling. In: BSAVA Manual of Canine Practice. Chapter 25:274-283. Available at:file:///C:/Users/Dr.Anand/Downloads/9781910443200.25.pdf.

MSD Veterinary manual. Aavilable at: https://www.msdvetmanual.com/dog-owners/digestive-disorders-of-dogs/disorders-of-the-stomach-and-intestines-in-dogs.

20

Cardiac Emergency

Mamta Mishra

Key Points

- Cardiac crises can result in deadly outcomes. Prompt and precise diagnosis leads to early symptom alleviation and increased survival.
- Many illnesses qualify as cardiac crises, including thromboembolic disease, cardiac tamponade, arrhythmogenic disease, and congestive heart failure.

Introduction

A cardiovascular emergency is defined as any condition affecting the heart or vasculature that prevents appropriate blood flow, tissue perfusion, or oxygenation. Cardiac emergencies include a wide range of disorders such as arrhythmias, cardiac tamponade/pericardial effusions, and congestive heart failure (CHF).

Arrhythmias

Arrhythmias can be associated with a wide range of disorders and cause clinical signs ranging from asymptomatic to collapse, depending on the arrhythmia's rate, frequency, and complexity, as well as the severity of cardiac dysfunction or other non-cardiac conditions.

1. Tachyarrhythmias are suspected on physical examination in critically sick patients on cardiac auscultation due to prolonged or paroxysmal bursts of tachycardia, typically at heart rates ranging from 150 to 300 beats per minute. Cardiac and noncardiac illnesses can cause either supraventricular or ventricular tachyarrhythmias. Noncardiac disease conditions such as sepsis, pancreatitis, autoimmune hemolytic anemia, pheochromocytoma, gastric-dilation-volvulus, splenic disease (e.g., neoplasia, torsion), and end-stage uremia can cause supraventricular and ventricular arrhythmias in the absence of structural heart disease. Myocardial ionic anomalies and arrhythmias can be brought on by electrolyte disturbances such as hypokalemia, hypocalcemia, hypomagnesemia, or hyperkalemia, as well as digoxin toxicity. Dilated

cardiomyopathy (DCM), infected endocarditis, myocarditis, severe congenital heart disease, progressive congestive heart failure due to DCM or mitral volvular disease (MVD), and cardiac neoplasia are other cardiac causes of tachyarrhythmias. Ventricular arrhythmias may also arise from traumatic myocarditis brought on by blunt chest trauma, which may be connected to myocardial bruising or ischemia-reperfusion injury. Based on the interpretation of the ECG, ventricular tachyarrhythmia is diagnosed. Ventricular arrhythmias that occur quickly (>150/min in dogs or >250/min in cats) or in prolonged runs (>30 seconds), are multiform, or occur extremely prematurely (the R-on-T phenomenon) are deemed to be more thermodynamically significant and potentially fatal. The severity of the arrhythmia, the underlying cause of the malfunction, and the hemodynamic state of the patients all influence the necessity and urgency of VT treatment. Certain ventricular arrhythmias would not need specialized antiarrhythmic treatment; instead, supportive measures including increasing oxygen supply, getting enough fluid and electrolyte therapy, and managing underlying medical conditions like sepsis or heart failure might be beneficial. Due to the possibility of side effects, injectable antiarrhythmic medication administration for the acute treatment of ventricular arrhythmias in cats presents challenges. Treatment suggestions for the acute management of severe and symptomatic canine ventricular arrhythmias include: a bolus of lidocaine intravenously (IV) ranging from 2-4 mg/kg is continued until the desired effect is achieved or an adverse effect is seen. A lidocaine CRI is started if the bolus injections are effective in reducing ventricular tachycardia (VT).

2. If lidocaine is ineffective, check that serum potassium and magnesium concentrations are sufficient. If not, consider slowly delivering IV procainamide boluses over a period of 3 to 5 minutes at doses of 2 to 8 mg/kg, up to a maximum of 16 mg/kg.
3. The following medications are advised for non-urgent ventricular arrhythmia management or oral maintenance therapy: doxiletine (4–8 mg/kg TID), amiodarone (10–20 mg/kg SID for up to 7–10 days, thereafter 5 mg/kg q24h SID), and tocainide (5–10 mg/kg TID).
4. Most dogs and cats that appear with atrial fibrillation in an emergency room have congestive heart failure (HF), which is treated with a combination of digoxin and diltiazem (described under congestive heart failure).
5. Most dogs and cats that appear with atrial fibrillation in an emergency room have congestive heart failure (HF), which is treated with a

combination of digoxin and diltiazem (described under congestive heart failure).

When a patient experiences occasional sinus arrest or a consistently slow heart rate, cardiac auscultation can be used to diagnose bradyarrhythmias. A heart rate of less than 60 beats per minute in dogs and less than 140 beats per minute in cats is commonly referred to as bradycardia. To differentiate between sinus bradycardia, high-grade AV block, atrial standstill, sinus node dysfunction, and either high-grade, second-degree AV block or total AV block, an ECG is required. The majority of animals that have bradyarrhythmias that are clinically significant exhibit syncope or weakness.

Bradyarrhythmia cases should be treated with atropine at 0.01 to 0.04 mg/kg IV or IM, glycopyrrolate at 0.005 to 0.01 mg/kg SC or IM, and terbutaline at 1.25 to 2.5 mg BID-TID.

Successful pacemaker implantations occur in healthy patients.

Cardiac tamponade/pericardial effusion

A physiological condition known as cardiac tamponade occurs when there is an increase in intrapericardial pressure due to pericardial effusion, which impairs ventricular filling and lowers cardiac output. Neoplasia, specifically right atrial hemangiosarcoma in large-breed dogs and chemodectomas (heart base tumors) in brachycephalic dogs, is the most frequent cause of pericardial effusion in elderly dogs.

Clinical signs

The symptoms include stomach distention, inappetence, coughing and retching, collapse, drowsiness, and intolerance to activity. Muffled heart sounds and tachycardia with weak, erratic pulses—known as pulse paradoxus—are noteworthy physical examination findings. When inspiration is accompanied by an unusually significant drop in systemic arterial pressure, this condition is known as pulse paradoxus. Heart tamponade has a strong correlation with pulse paradoxus. Physical examination findings include hepatosplenomegaly, ascites, pale mucous membranes, poor capillary refill time, and jugular venous distention.

Diagnosis

Radiography, echocardiography, and ECG are advised.

Treatment

The only therapy that can effectively relieve cardiac tamponade right away is pericardiocentesis. Combining diuretics and vasodilators with other medications can potentially be hazardous as they decrease ventricular filling and result in hypotension. While the pericardiocentesis is being prepared, it is advisable to place a peripheral IV catheter and administer IV fluids to increase cardiac output. It is advisable to monitor for potential re-effusion following the centesis, particularly in dogs suspected of having hemangiosarcoma.

Congestive Heart Failure

Heart failure is not a particular illness or condition. This syndrome occurs when the cardiovascular system experiences severe malfunction and is unable to sustain proper blood circulation. The cardiovascular system can be compromised by heart disease through a few distinct and restricted processes. Therefore, heart failure can only cause a limited number of distinct symptoms to appear.

Blood buildup in the body's major organs, usually the lungs, but occasionally other organs, results in congestive heart failure. This can cause aberrant organ function, fluid enlargement, or both.

Clinical Signs

The causes of heart failure and the afflicted heart chamber determine the symptoms of heart failure. The symptoms of left-sided congestive heart failure are linked to a pressure buildup in the blood vessels that supply the left ventricle. As a result, fluid builds up in the lungs (pulmonary edema). The most typical symptoms are coughing, dyspnea, and exercise intolerance, which is exhaustion accompanied by dyspnea during physical activity. Lack of blood flow and oxygen to the brain causes many dogs with congestive heart failure on the left side to pass out. They might also collapse and have low blood pressure and heart rate. Compared to healthy dogs, dogs with left-side congestive heart failure frequently breathe more quickly.

Increased blood pressure in the body's veins and capillaries, as well as the vessels supplying blood to the right atrium, is a consequence of right-sided congestive heart failure. This could result in fluid accumulation in the limbs, liver, chest cavity, and belly (ascites).

Treatment

In order to enhance cardiac muscle function, regulate arrhythmias and blood pressure, enhance blood flow, and lessen the volume of blood filling the heart prior to contraction, heart failure must be treated. If left unchecked, any of these can worsen damage to the heart and blood vessels. Reducing the volume of fluid in the chest cavity, abdomen, or lungs is also essential.

For the treatment of fluid overload in animals, diuretics (furosemide 2 to 4 mg/kg IV or IM; spironolactone 1 to 2 mg/kg PO q24h with meals; torsemide 0.2 to 0.4 mg/kg PO q24h) are typically administered. Pimobendan enhances cardiac output, dilates blood vessels, improves heart muscle contraction, and lowers diastolic pressure when taken orally (0.2 to 0.3 mg/kg PO q12h, empty stomach). Digoxin (0.002 to 0.005 mg/kg PO q12h), a member of the class of medications known as positive inotropes, is prescribed to patients who have specific arrhythmias in order to help the heart muscle contract.

Vasodilators (Hydralazine at 0.5 to 3 mg/kg IV bolus q12h or as a CRI at 1.5 to 5 mcg/kg/min IV; Nitroglycerine 2% ointment ¼ inch/5 kg TID topically for the first 24h) and ACE inhibitors (Enalapril and Benazepril 0.25 to 0.5 mg/kg PO every 12–24h) can dilate blood vessels, which lowers blood pressure. In certain cases of congestive heart failure, beta-blockers such as dopamine (1–15 mcg/kg/min in CRI), dobutamine (2–15 mcg/kg/min CRI), and calcium channel blockers (Diltiazem at 0.1 to 0.2 mg/kg IV slowly; amlodipine 0.1–0.2 mg/Kg SID-BID) can be beneficial.

It's possible that dogs with pulmonary edema, or fluid in the lungs, and severe left-sided congestive heart failure won't obtain enough oxygen. oxygen supplementation through the use of a nose tube, oxygen cage, oxygen collar, or tight mask. Patients with chronic airway illness are typically the only ones eligible for bronchodilator therapy (10 mg/kg/6-8h for dogs and 4 mg/kg/8-12h for cats; 11 mg/kg/8h for dogs and 5–6 mg/kg/12h for cats). Treatment for congestive heart failure is not common. This does not apply to dogs that pass out due to a transient cardiac arrhythmia linked to heart illness.

Because they can exacerbate the underlying fluid in the lungs, cough suppressants are generally not advised in the treatment of congestive heart failure. However, if a dog with serious heart disease is coughing and an X-ray of the chest indicates that there is no fluid in the lungs, the coughing may be the result of chronic bronchitis, a long-term inflammation of the airways. For certain pets, cough suppressants might be beneficial. When congestive heart failure is causing a respiratory crisis in a dog that is having severe breathing difficulties, anti-anxiety medications may be given judiciously to help the dog calm down.

A needle is introduced into the chest cavity or the abdomen, respectively, during thoracentesis and abdominocentesis, two surgical procedures used to remove excess fluid. Dogs with congestive heart failure who have fluid buildup in these places may benefit from treatment with it.

Nourishment

For animals suffering from heart failure, maintaining a salt balance, decreasing inflammation, providing enough calories, and making up for any nutrients that are lacking are the general nutritional objectives. Omega-3 fatty acid supplements may help control arrhythmias and reduce inflammation. When standard treatment is ineffective for dogs with severe congestive heart failure, a low-sodium diet is often advised.

Omega-3 fatty acid supplementation is helpful for CHF patients in humans, and it is probably good for dogs as well, particularly if cardiac cachexia is present. It has been proposed to take 40 mg/kg of eicosapentaenoic acid (EPA) and 25 mg/kg of docosahexaenoic acid (DHA) orally every 24 hours. Supplementing with taurine and carnitine has been recommended, and it might be suitable for people with impaired systolic function.

Cardio-Pulmonary *Resuscitation*

When an animal has cardiopulmonary arrest (CPA), it is necessary to administer cardiopulmonary resuscitation (CPR). The goal of CPR is to keep the brain and other essential organs supplied with enough blood and oxygen to sustain life until more sophisticated medical treatment can be initiated. The following are suggested CPR techniques for cats and dogs: Until endotracheal intubation and positive-pressure breathing with 100% oxygen can be achieved, mouth-to-nose resuscitation should be carried out. In mouth-to-nose breathing, the ratio of compression to ventilation should be 30:2. Ventilation should be administered at a rate of 10 breaths per minute (1 breath every 6 seconds), with a volume of 10 mL/kg and an inspiratory duration of one second, as soon as the airway has been established. These breaths should ideally come with a portable bag-valve-mask device.

In tiny animals, external chest compression should be used in conjunction with ventilation to enhance circulation. Important considerations when doing chest compressions are as follows:

- The animal is put in lateral recumbency (or, in the case of animals with barrel-chested chests, dorsal recumbency).
- Regardless of the animal's size, compressions should be administered rapidly, compressing 1/3 to 1/2 of the thoracic wall's width and allowing for full recoil in between.
- Compressions should be performed over the widest part of the thorax or directly over the heart (at the fourth and fifth intercostal spaces) at a rate of 100–120 compressions per minute.

References

DeFrancesco. (2013). Management of Cardiac Emergencies in Small Animals.Vet Clin Small Anim 43: 817–842

Sudan, N.A. and Bhawal, M.S. (2009). Miscellaneous disease conditions. In: Textbook of Veterinary Medicine. Sharma, MC., Mahesh Kumar and Sharma, R.D. (Ed.), ICAR, Krishi Anusandhan Bhavan, Pusa, New Delhi. PP:599-601,

The Merck veterinary manual. Whitehouse Station, NJ :Merck & Co., Inc.

21

Eye Emergency

Kumari Chandrakala

The diagnosis of blindness is as follows: an animal that is blind is apprehensive, easily agitated, has an uptight head position with a feeling gait, stumbles forward, steps up high, collides with obstacles in its path, and lacks the cross reflex, photomotor pupillary reflex, and palpebral reflex.

Clinical examination of the eye:

- By necked eye
- By magnifying lenses
- By catoptric test: use to detect opacities of the cornea and lens
- By ophthalmoscope
- By tonometry: use to measure intraocular pressure.

Chalazion/ tarsal gland cyst.

Hordeolum/stye: localize inflammatory swelling of eye lashes due to staphylococcus.

Dacro-adenitis: inflammation of the lacrimal gland.

Blepharitis : inflammation of the eyelids.

Trichiasis : eyelashes are directed slightly inward.

Districhiasis : congenital condition in which two rows of eyelashes are present and the inner row causes irritation to the conjunctiva.

Ptosis: dropping of the upper eyelid due to paralysis of the seventh cranial nerve.

Lagophthalmos: inomplete closure of the eye.

Blepharospasm : partial or complete closure of the eyelid.

Ectropion:

Enteropion :

Exophthalmos/Proptosis : an abnormal protrusion of the eye ball.

Endopthalmos/ pig eye

Hyphema : hemorrhage in anterior chamber of eye.

Diseases of Eye

1. ***Hydropthalmos:*** an increase in the aqueous humor of the eyeball raises intraocular pressure, which in turn causes the eyeball to grow because the tunics become weaker. typical in calf cattle.
2. ***Glaucoma:*** marked increase in intraocular pressure brought on by an excessive amount of aqueous humor (caused by either decreased or increased synthesis of drainase) without an increase in the size of the eye ball. Typical in canines.

Theileriosis, cataract, and lens luxation are the causes.

Symptoms: Exophthalmos and lagopthalmos are caused by the eye-ball bulging forward as a result of a general increase in fluid contents. Blepharospasm, blindness, and lacrimation. Lack of or slow corneal reflex.

Diagnosis using tonometry or digital palpation.

Treatment: 2% PILOCARPINE eye drops, applied once daily.

- Applying a 0.25% or 5% TIMOLOL eye drop once a day.
- Diuretics (1g/kg IV mannitol)
- Low water intake; • Laxative diet; • Salt-free diet.

3. ***Keratoconjunctivitis*** is an inflammation of the conjunctiva and cornea concurrently.

Causes include injury, irritants, fungal, viral, and bacterial infections.

Symptoms include redness, swelling, lacrimation, cloudiness of the cornea, photophobia, blepharospasm, and, in the case of a chronic illness, blindness and corneal opacity, depending on the type of invasive pathogen.

diagnosis using an opthalmoscope and an ocular discharge test in a lab.

Treatment:

- Eye washing with M/E and NSS.
- Eye drops with a broad-spectrum antibiotic (5-7 drops, BID for 5-7 days).
- For non-ulcerative eye reasons, a broad-spectrum antibiotic and steroid eye drop may be given at 5-7 drops BID, for 5-7 days.

Weekly intravenous vitamin A injections or daily oral preparations are to be administered as supportive therapy.

4. **Cataract**

- The lens's total or partial opacity.
- Surgery is necessary to correct the problem; medication is ineffective.

22

Ear Emergency

Mamta Mishra

Key Points

- The most frequent physical damage in animals is an aural hematoma;
- Otitis externa is known to result in Zepp's operation, or drainboard from the lateral ear wall.

Introduction

An alternative name for the ear is the sensory organ of hearing. It could display both functional issues and structural abnormalities.

Anatomical abnormalities

Diseases of Pinna

The pinna is affected by several dermatological disorders. In rare cases, a disease only first affects the pinna or the pinna alone. A diagnosis is best determined based on the findings of a comprehensive history, a full physical and dermatologic examination, and the thoughtful selection and assessment of certain diagnostic tests, as with any dermatologic disorder.

Arthropod Bite Pinnal/Aural Dermatitis

Pinnae dermatitis is frequently brought on by arthropods, either directly by the parasite's bite or indirectly through hypersensitivity. Ticks can irritate the pinna or the canal inside the ear, depending on where they are attached. The external ear canals of horses, cattle, sheep, goats, deer, rabbits, cats, and dogs are parasitized by the spinous ear tick (Otobius megnini), which is found in the southwest United States, south and central America, southern Africa, and India.

Clinical signs

Head shaking, head rubbing, or drooped pinnae.

Treatment

It affects the animal as well as the surroundings when it comes to large animals. After using forceps to mechanically remove as many ticks as possible, the coat should be sprayed or dipped with acaricide. Diazinon, pyrethroids, carbaryls, and avermectins (ivermectin, doramectin, and eprinomectin) are a few options for insecticides. These products can be poured on or applied with a high-pressure sprayer. Long-term acaricide use can lead to pollution in the environment and the selection of resistant ticks.

As an eco-friendly substitute for acaracides, vaccines have demonstrated some efficacy against tick infestations in Australia, Cuba, Mexico, and other Latin American nations; however, they are not able to entirely eradicate the infestation or the spread of pathogens carried by ticks. In the USA, these vaccines are not currently accessible.

Auricular Hematomas in Dogs, Cats and Pigs

In dogs, cats, and pigs, auricular hematomas are small to large, fluid-filled swellings that form on the concave surface of the pinnae (Fig. 22.1). The trauma from shaking one's head or scratching one's ears because of itching is the pathophysiology of the lesions' development. The ear canals are the main locations of allergic inflammation, itching, and secondary infection in dogs with atopic dermatitis and food allergies.

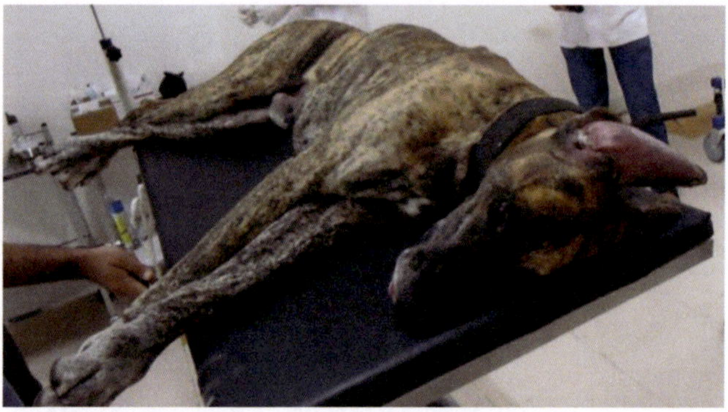

Fig. 22.1. Aural hematoma in a male Great Dane dog.

Treatment

Surgical drainage is the course of treatment. Upon emptying and cleaning, a few mattress stitches can be inserted to close the "pocket." In around 50% of cases, drainage and glucocorticoid instillation are successful. Using an IV catheter or a butterfly connection is the best way to achieve drainage. To fill the hole without producing skin distension, glucocorticoids are injected. Often, this treatment is combined with a brief course of oral glucocorticoids at a low anti-inflammatory dosage. To stop a recurrence, the underlying issue must be addressed.

Diseases of External Ear canal

Otitis Externa

Distal to the tympanic membrane, otitis externa is an inflammation of the external ear canal; the ear pinna may or may not be affected. It is among the most frequent causes of small animal (particularly dog) veterinarian visits. Otitis externa can manifest as unilateral or bilateral, acute or chronic. It is rare in large animals and commonly observed in rabbits, where it is thought to be caused by the mite *Psoroptes cuniculi.*

Primary causes

The following are the main causes: foreign bodies, fungal (Aspergillus), viral (Distemper), autoimmune/immune-mediated (Pemphigus foliaceus, vasculitis, etc.), allergy, parasites (*Otodectes, Demodex, Sarcoptes*), endocrine disease (hypothyroidism, hyperadrenocorticism), epithelialization disorders (sebaceous adenitis, zinc-responsive dermatitis), fungal (Aspergillus), viral (Distemper), and miscellaneous (proliferative necrotizing otitis of cats, juvenile cellulitis).

Otitis externa secondary causes result in abnormal ear illness. When the underlying cause is ignored, these issues can become persistent or recurrent. Secondary causes include yeast (*Malassezia*), medication responses, overcleaning, and bacteria (*Staphylococcus, Streptococcus, Enterococcus, Pseudomonas, Proteus*, etc.).

Diagnosis

Following a thorough physical examination and dermatological assessment, the ears should be inspected, starting with the least damaged or bothersome ones. Sedation or systemic glucocorticoids may be necessary in really painful patients for a few days before an otoscopic examination. The pinna and ear canals can be palpated to detect the presence of discomfort, mineralization (from chronicity), and edema. Individuals who have significant, long-term alterations in their ear canals may require more sophisticated ear imaging. It is important to assess the pinnae for exudate presence, lichenification, ulceration, crusting, erosion, and erythema. Pinnae can be sampled by dermatophyte culture, mineral oil preparations (*Demodex, Sarcoptes*), skin scrapes, or surface cytology (yeast, bacteria, and inflammatory cells).

Otoscopic evaluation should be performed on all dermatologic patients, if possible

The canal should be examined for lumps, glandular hyperplasia, erythema, erosion or ulceration, stenosis, and exudate (quantity and quality). Examining the tympanic membrane for bulging, rupture, or color changes should be done whenever possible. However, because of the exudate in the horizontal canal, the membrane is frequently invisible, necessitating cleaning or flushing. Prior to doing any cleaning, samples (cytology, mineral oil preparations) should be taken. When proliferative tissues impede proper visualization of the tympanic membrane, when otitis media is suspected of being the source of relapsing bacterial otitis externa, and when neurologic symptoms coexist with otitis externa, radiography of the osseous bullae is required. Proliferative or lytic osseous alterations, along with fluid densities, are frequently indicative of middle ear involvement. Regrettably, in a large number of otitis media cases, radiographs are normal. When adequate treatment fails to alleviate severe, chronic otitis media, a CT or MRI scan, if one is available, should be conducted. On CT or MRI scans, there may be signs of fluid in the middle ear in some clinically normal dogs.

Treatment

Otitis externa can be successfully treated with owner compliance, inflammation control, targeted antibiotic therapy, and an underlying cause investigation. Owners must set realistic expectations and be aware that treating or improving otitis externa may take some time.Many patients first need their discomfort and/or itching to be managed. Glucocorticoids lessen pain, edema, and inflammation, which eventually improves the owner's capacity to properly care for and clean the ears at home. Most frequently, prednisone and triamcinolone are utilized; the length and dosage of each medication are determined by the severity and chronicity of the ailment. The owner should, if at all feasible, watch while the veterinarian does the initial ear cleaning. The kind of infection or exudate present will determine which ear cleaning is best, but it's crucial that the cleaner has a neutral pH to minimize discomfort in inflamed ears and an enticing scent to boost owner compliance. Cleaning infected ears with thick, dry, or waxy debris two or three times a week using a ceruminolytic solution such as dioctyl sodium sulfosuccinate (DSS) or carbamide peroxide may be necessary. It may be necessary to clean infected ears with abundant purulent discharge once or twice a day. Squalene should be included in the ear cleaner if rods are observed, as Pseudomonas may be the reason. This bacteria can create a biofilm that shields microorganisms from antibiotics. Rinse the ears well with warm water to get rid of any remaining ear cleanser. Detergents and DSS should not be used if the tympanic membrane is torn; instead, the ear should be flushed with milder cleansers such as saline, saline plus povidone iodine, or Tris EDTA.

Effective treatment may involve topical and systemic antibacterial and anti-inflammatory medications in addition to cleansing. Depending on the diagnosis, the course of treatment could last anywhere from seven to ten days to several months.

Diseases of Internal Ear canal

Otitis media and interna

Dogs, cats, rabbits, ruminants, horses, pigs, and camelids are among the small and large domestic animals that can suffer from otitis media, an infection of the middle ear structures. Animals of various ages may be affected, and it may be unilateral or bilateral. Otitis media is typically caused by pharyngeal bacteria migrating into the auditory tube or by an infection spreading from the external ear canal through the tympanic membrane. There are times when an infection travels through the hematogenous route or from the inner ear to the middle ear. If left untreated, otitis media can result in rupture of an intact tympanic membrane, which can cause ottorrhea, or otitis externa, or otitis interna, which is inflammation of the inner ear structures.

Clinical signs

Otitis externa (head shaking, discharge, ear canal inflammation), Horner syndrome, facial nerve paralysis or palsy, kerato-conjunctivitis sicca, and diminished hearing are among the clinical manifestations of otitis media. While it does happen, otitis media is less prevalent in cats than in dogs.

Head tilt, circling or incoordination, and spontaneous horizontal or rotating nystagmus are among the clinical signs of otitis interna. The vestibule-cochlear nerve (cranial nerve VIII) is compromised by inflammation in otitis interna, leading to peripheral vestibular disease symptoms like head tilt or circling, leaning or falling towards the affected side, general incoordination, or spontaneous horizontal nystagmus with the fast phase away from the affected side. As a result, hearing loss occurs. Listeriosis is a common differential diagnosis for otitis media/interna in ruminants. Animals with listeriosis are typically sad, but other cranial nerves besides VII and VIII may also be impacted, leading to symptoms including dysphagia or a lack of facial sensibility.

Diagnosis

A thorough medical history, a physical examination that identifies relevant clinical indicators, and, if practical, an otoscopic examination that verifies a bulging or irregular tympanic membrane are the first steps in diagnosing otitis media/interna. Tympanic membrane otoscopic examination may be restricted because of stenosis, ear canal structure, exudate, or environmental or animal restrictions. Tympanic membrane abnormalities can enlarge, thicken, turn opaque, or burst. The dorsal portion of the tympanic membrane contains the pars flaccida, which can enlarge when there is an increase in pressure from soft tissue, fluid, or air. Nonetheless, in certain instances of otitis media, the tympanic membrane may appear normal or intact, and some animals that are normally do not have air-caused bulging. While video otoscopy can aid in improving tympanic membrane visualization, it is challenging to observe the middle ear without a tiny arthroscope.

Compared to standard radiographs, advanced imaging methods (such as CT or MRI) are more sensitive. Changes seen on CT or MRI scans include the bulla's wall thickening, sclerosis, and lysis, in addition to the bulla itself being filled with soft tissue or fluid.

Treatment

If the tympanic membrane is intact, a myringotomy, middle ear flushing, inflammation control, and treatment of underlying illnesses or infections are all possible options.

Otorrhoea

An infectious agent has caused a painful inflammation of the external ear canal's skin, accompanied by drainage. On rare occasions, it is observed during a distemper episode due to certain unidentified constitutional variables (eczematous otorrhoea), excessive sebum and ceruminous gland secretion, and glandular buildup.

Clinical signs and symptoms

The animal displays signs of discomfort by shaking its head, rubbing its ears against the walls and floors, and scratching. There is an unpleasant-smelling, purulent discharge coming from the ear. The head may be tilted to the affected side if only one ear is impacted. Chronic cases might exhibit hypertrophic changes and vegetation obstructing the ear canal, which results in deafness.

Treatment

Hair cutting, medicated soap and water cleaning of the surrounding area, hydrogen peroxide, methylated spirit, potassium permanganate (1:1000), zinc sulfate lotion (1-2%), and ear canal cleaning are all part of the treatment. using the appropriate ear drops and applying antibiotic ointment topically in accordance with the findings of the sensitivity and culture tests.

Functional Abnormalities

Deafness

Reduced hearing and no sense of sound are typical in dogs and cats, and to a lesser degree in other animals. There are two types of deafness: sensorineural or conductive, congenital or later onset, and hereditary or acquired. In dogs and cats, congenital and hereditary deafness most frequently results from white pigmentation. The most common conditions affecting adult and elderly animals include presbycusis, noise shock, medication toxicity, and otitis media.

References

Singh J., Singh S., and Tyagi, RPS (2019). The Special sense organs: Ruminant Surgery: A Textbook of the Surgical Diseases of Cattle, Buffaloes, Camels, Sheep and Goats [CBS Publishers & Distributors]: pp 549-572

Slatter DH. (2003). Ear: Textbook of Small Animal Surgery [Saunders], Vol 2: 1737-1767

23

Gastro-Intestinal Emergency

Mamta Mishra

Key Points

- Neurologic dysfunction, which can show up as a wide range of perplexing symptoms and indicators, can accompany gastrointestinal disorders that cause malabsorption and the ensuing nutritional deficits.
- Digestive illnesses are among the most common problems in animals living in tropical countries. They often manifest as intestinal blockage, malabsorption, malnourishment, bleeding in the gastrointestinal tract, diarrhea, and stomach pain or distention.

Introduction

Animal digestive problems can be brought on by a range of conditions, including infections, parasites, and other illnesses. In older dogs and cats, gastrointestinal (GI) disorders of the alimentary tract and hepatobiliary system are prevalent. The majority of the time, GI symptoms in affected animals are caused by inflammatory illnesses; however, degenerative lesions and motility issues can also occur. Acute and chronic conditions are two general classifications for gastrointestinal diseases. Dietary errors, or the worsening of long-term gastrointestinal disorders, are the most frequent causes of acute gastrointestinal disorders. Alongside chronic gastrointestinal disease, colitis or inflammatory bowel disease are frequently diagnosed.

Choke/Esophageal Obstruction

Choking occurs when food particles or other objects lodge in the esophagus. The crops that are most hampered by animals are grain, apples, beets, potatoes, turnips, corn stalks, ears of corn, or hay. Animals recuperating from a general anesthetic or prolonged pharmacological restraint may occasionally exhibit choking or esophageal obstruction symptoms.

Clinical Indications

Horses with dysphagia, ptyalism, coughing, or nasal discharge of feed material or saliva are clinical signs of oesophageal obstruction. The horse may display signs of nervousness or retch by extending and arching its neck. Horses that are afflicted might keep eating or drinking, which would exacerbate their clinical signs.

Ptyalism, nasal discharge of food and drink, and free-gas bloat are examples of clinical signs in cattle. Ruminants can exhibit ptyalism, bruxism, tongue protrusion, head extension, bloating and distress. They can also be recumbent. Since complete and acute esophageal blockage might result in asphyxia, it needs to be treated as an emergency.

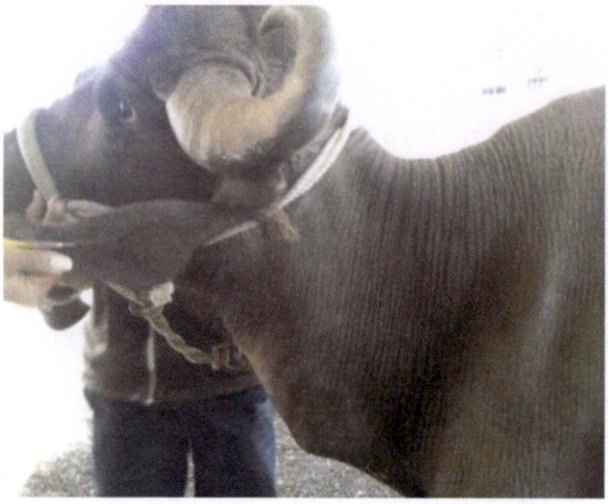

Fig. 23.1. Esophageal obstruction (bulged area at ventral neck) in a female Jaffarabadi buffalo.

(*Source*: Kumar et al. (2016). Ultrasonographic, radiographic diagnosis and management of esophageal obstruction in Jaffarabadi buffaloes and Gir cattle. Buffalo Bulletin 35(4): 549-556)

Diagnosis

- Based on clinical indications;
- Results of oro- or nasogastric tube insertion;
- Endoscopy

Treatment

- Oro- or nasogastric tube passage to ease esophageal blockage;
- Sedatives and muscle relaxants to relax the esophagus;

Drugs that are antimicrobial and anti-inflammatory

When feed and water are stopped, many esophageal blockages in horses clear on their own. With spontaneous resolve, sedatives (such as detomidine and xylazine) can be helpful. Oxytocin (0.11-0.22 U/kg, IV, once) is useful in relaxing the smooth muscle of the esophagus. Any horse suspected of having an esophageal obstruction should have an endoscopic examination or a nasogastric tube inserted to ensure that the obstruction has completely disappeared. When conservative therapy fails to provide the desired results, esophageal lavage should be administered to horses in the following order: A nasogastric tube should be inserted up to the level of the obstruction after IV sedation. To wash the esophagus, a stomach pump sends water to the obstruction location and gradually inserts and removes the tube. When there are clinical signs of discomfort, esophageal obstruction with bloat in cattle is considered an emergency, and bloat must be alleviated by trocarization through the left sublumbar fossa. Once the tympany has been relieved, solid things (potatoes, for example) may rub themselves free or come loose on their own since saliva softens their outer surfaces. Ruminant choking may be treated by standing esophageal lavage administered through an orogastric tube. It is often possible to drive large foreign bodies into the rumen without any further difficulties. In rare instances of esophageal obstruction brought on by foreign objects, esophagotomy may be necessary. Common antimicrobials used in animals recovering from choking include trimethoprim and sulfamethoxazole (30 mg/kg, PO, every 12 hours), procaine penicillin G (22,000 U/kg, IM, every 6–12 hours), and potassium penicillin G (2.6 mg/kg, IV or IM, every 6–12 hours). Anaerobic infections can be effectively treated with metronidazole (15 mg/kg, PO every 6 hours). NSAIDs are often only given in the acute phase (the first few days) and only with caution due to the risk of gastrointestinal and renal adverse effects, especially in horses who are already dehydrated. The most often used anti-inflammatory drugs in these situations are phenylbutazone (2.2–4.4 mg/kg, PO or IV, every 12 hours) and flunixin meglumine (1.1 mg/kg, IV, every 12 hours).

Colic

- Any abdominal pain can be classified as colic, although horse owners often refer to colic as gastrointestinal problems. Horse colic has several underlying causes, but they are all related to the anatomy and microbiology of the gastrointestinal tract. Some of the more common causes of colic are: diets heavy in grains and deficient in forages Moldy or contaminated feed
- Sudden shift in feed
- Infestation of parasites
- Inadequate water consumption, resulting in impaction colic
- Ingestion of sand
- Prolonged usage of NSAIDS
- Anxiety
- Dental issues

Clinical signs

Signs of colic include:

- Absence of gut sounds
- Looking at sides
- Biting or kicking flank
- Pawing the ground or air
- Laying down and/or rolling
- Faecal balls small, dry, or not produced
- Poor appetite
- Change in drinking behaviour
- Increased heart rate
- Abnormal breathing
- Sweating, restlessness
- Dullness or lethargy
- Tacky or dry gums
- Abnormal coloured gums

Treatment

Fluid deficit	**% dehydration × body weight (kg)**	**4%–10% × 500 = 20–50 L**
Maintenance	50 mL/kg/24 h	50 × 500 = 25 L/24 h
Fluid losses	Estimate reflux or diarrhea volume	-
Rate of administration	50% in 1–2 h; 50% throughout rest of day	20–35 L in first 1–2 h; remainder distributed throughout next 23 h
Bicarbonate deficit	0-3 x Bodyweight x Base deficit (mmol) (kg) (mmol/litre)	-

In situations of colic, nonsteroidal anti-inflammatory medications are utilized to reduce pain and inflammation. 2.2 to 4.4 mg/kg IV of phenylbutazone, 0.25 to 1.1 mg/kg IV of flunixin meglumine, 1.2 to 2.2 mg/kg IV of ketoprofen, 0.2 to 1.1 mg/kg IV of xylazine, 0.03 to 0.1 mg/kg IV or IM of Acepromazine, 0.3 to 0.66 mg/kg IV or IM of Morphine, 2.0 mg/kg IM of Pethidine, 0.05 to 0.075 mg/kg bdy wt. IV of Butorphanol, and 0.3 to 0.6 mg/kg IV of Pentazocine.

Spasmolytics can reduce pain associated with an increased frequency of intestinal contractions or intraluminal obstructions such as impactions. Horses with colic should not be treated with atropine. You can also use hyoscine at 0.3 mg/kg bdy with a gradual IV.

Mineral oil (5–10 ml/kg) can be given once or twice a day; a 5% solution of dioctyl sodium sulfosuccinate (10–20 mg/kg) can be given every 48 hours; and psyllium hydrophilic mucilloid (1 g/kg) can be given orally through nasogastric tubes up to four times a day.

Hospital or surgical care may be necessary if the horse does not get well after taking medication or undergoing treatments on the farm. In order to identify and perhaps treat the source of the horse's colic symptoms, abdominal exploratory surgery is performed while the animal is under general anesthesia for colic surgery.

Prevention of Colic in Horses

The chances of developing colic can be minimized by following these tips:

- Make sure your pet has access to clean water at all times.
- Provide pasture turnout.
- Steer clear of feeding on the ground in sandy regions.
- Offer grain and pelleted feed only when absolutely necessary.
- Keep an eye out for any signs of colic, particularly during feeding, exercise, or schedule adjustments.
- Regular deworming programs and fecal egg counts, as advised by veterinarians, are important methods of preventing parasites.
- Monitor any horses that have experienced colic in the past, broodmares in the first two months following foaling, and horses on nonsteroidal anti-inflammatories like flunixine meglumine.

Tympany (Bloat)

Bloat is a common digestive ailment in ruminants. The disease is characterized by gas buildup in the rumen and reticulum, the first two stomach chambers in ruminants, and it can impair the animal's ability to breathe and digest food. Both frothy and free-gas bloat, which can occur in calves raised on pasture or in confinement, are commonly recognized forms of the disease. Free-gas bloat is characterized by its quick onset and high mortality rate, even though it is less common than foamy bloat. The most frequent associations are with heart or oesophageal blockage. The most common treatments for free-gas bloating involve either clearing the esophageal blockage or passing a tube through the esophagus and into the rumen. Foathy bloat is caused by gas released during the fermentation of easily digested meals being trapped. A stable foam that is created during fermentation prevents the eructation of fermentation gas. Tubing is essentially unhelpful in treating frothy-bloat because froth prevents gas from being distributed from the pressurized rumen via the tube to the atmosphere.

Clinical Signs

Cattle with bloat may display the following signs:

The patient may exhibit the following symptoms:

- a distended left belly,
- inability to graze,
- reluctance to move,
- distressed appearance (vocalize, eyes bulging),
- difficulty urinating and defecating, rapid breathing, and an open mouth with a protruding tongue.
- Stagging Under extreme conditions, the animal will pass out.
- Quick mortality results from the rumen's bloated state compressing the lungs, obstructing breathing and tissue oxygenation, and reducing blood flow.

Treatment

Extremely bloated and anxious animals need to be helped right away. To do this, a wide-bore trocar and cannula are inserted into the left side's rumen (the area with the highest swelling). A trochar and cannula will typically not be sufficient to relieve pressure in situations with foamy bloat; instead, a 10–20 cm incision made with a clean, sharp knife would be necessary. To lessen foamy bloat, more antifoaming chemicals are added.Doses of 250–500 mL are effective for several antifoaming substances, including mineral oils (paraffins) and vegetable oils (such as peanut, corn, and soybean).

Surfactant dioctyl sodium sulfosuccinate is sold as a proprietary anti-bloat treatment (1,000 mg, PO by stomach tube or drench, every 24 hours as needed). It is typically paired with one of the following oils. Legume-induced bloat can be effectively treated with poloxalene (25–50 g PO as a drench, if needed for emergency treatment of ruminal tympany in cattle), but not feedlot-induced bloat.(Minimum withholding of 48 hours). Additionally, the frothy debris in the rumen is manually scraped out using antifoaming chemicals (40 mL of a 50% solution of alcohol ethoxylate and pluronic detergents, PO intraruminally 1 hour before feeding, every 24 hours).

Control and Prevention

Steering clear of pasture bloat is not always simple. Feeding hay, particularly orchard grass, prior to sending cattle out on pasture, maintaining grass dominance in the sward, or restricting intake via strip grazing—in which animals move to a new strip in the afternoon as opposed to the early morning—

all help reduce the risk of bloat. Hay should make up at least one-third of the diet in order to effectively lower the risk of bloating. When the pasture is in the pre-bloom stage and the bloat danger is high, feeding hay or strip grazing may be dependable; however, these strategies are less dependable when the pasture is in the pre-bloom stage and the bloat potential is high.

Compared to established pastures, bloat is more likely in immature or rapidly expanding grasslands.

Gastritis or Gastroenteritis

The illness known as "gastritis" is a general name for vomiting that can occur suddenly or repeatedly due to inflammation of the stomach mucosa.

Causes

Endoparasitism (e.g., Physaloptera sp [dog, cat], Ollulanus sp [cat]), viral infection (e.g., canine parvovirus gastroenteritis, feline panleukopenia), systemic illness (e.g., pancreatitis, uremic gastropathy, hypoadrenocorticism), dietary indiscretion (e.g., ingestion of foreign material or novel, spoiled, or contaminated foods), drug or toxin ingestion (e.g., antibiotics, NSAIDs, corticosteroids, plants, chemicals), etc.

Clinical signs

It is common to experience abrupt vomiting along with bile, food, froth, blood (frank or digested), or signs of something being consumed (such as grass, bones, foreign material, etc.). The intensity, frequency, and underlying reason for vomiting determine other clinical signs.

Diagnosis

A diagnosis is based on a thorough history, clinical findings, and the patient's reaction to symptomatic treatment. When cranial abdominal discomfort is present, dogs may assume a "praying" posture. A CBC, serum biochemical profile, and urinalysis may be followed by more specialist clinic pathologic testing. Abdominal ultrasonography and/or radiography with plain or barium contrast may be advised.

Treatment

Treatment is typically supportive and symptomatic. Oral fluids can often be given in small amounts, with the volume increasing as the vomiting stops. Ice, either crushed or in cube form, can serve as the only source of water initially. Subcutaneous infusion of a balanced electrolyte solution that is isotonic may be sufficient to correct mild fluid deficiency (5%). A more comprehensive diagnostic diagnosis is necessary if the animal's clinical condition requires

IV fluid therapy or if the dehydration is moderate to severe. For a period of 12 to 24 hours, oral intake should be avoided if the vomiting is severe. A commercially available prescription diet or small portions of a bland, low-fat, easily digestible meal (such as boiled lean beef, chicken, or cottage cheese and rice) could be added frequently, with a gradual transition to the 3 diet in 5 days. Common antiemetics include maropitant (1 mg/kg, SC or IV, every 24 hours; or 2 mg/kg, PO, every 24 hours up to 5 days) and ondansetron (0.1–1 mg/kg, PO or IV, every 12–24 hours). Another alternative is to use metoclopramide (0.2–0.5 mg/kg, IM, SC, or PO, every 6–8 hours; or 5–20 mcg/kg as a constant-rate infusion). If there is a confirmed or suspected GI blockage, it is not advised.

Gastrointestinal protectants such as H2-receptor antagonists (famotidine, for example, at 0.5–1 mg/kg, PO, SC, IM, or IV, every 12–24 hours) or proton pump inhibitors (omeprazole, at 0.5–1.5 mg/kg, PO, every 12–24 hours; or pantoprazole, at 1 mg/kg, IV, every 12 hours) may be indicated if gastric ulceration is confirmed or highly suspected. In addition to symptomatic treatment and dietary modifications, immunosuppressive medicine is frequently needed for animals with moderate to severe illnesses that have been histologically confirmed sick. Starting at 2 mg/kg/day, PO (cats and small dogs) or 40–50 mg/m2 (medium to large dogs), prednisone (or prednisolone in cats) is gradually lowered to the lowest effective dose for controlling clinical symptoms.An additional immunosuppressive agent (azathioprine at 2 mg/kg, PO, every 24-48 hours, or cyclosporine at 5 mg/kg, PO, every 12 hours; cats: chlorambucil at 2 mg [total dose], PO, every 48-72 hours for 2-4 weeks, then tapered to 2 mg every 72-96 hours) may be considered if clinical signs persist despite dietary changes and prednisone therapy.

Gastric Dilation and Volvolus (GDV)

Large and gigantic breed dogs are mostly affected by the potentially fatal disease known as gastric dilatation and volvulus, or GDV. Quick surgical and medical attention is required to improve the patient's prognosis.

Etiology

Breeds at risk for GDV include the Great Dane, German Shepherd, Irish Setter, Gordon Setter, Weimaraner, Saint Bernard, Standard Poodle, and Bassett Hound. There is no sex predisposition, and older dogs seem to be more vulnerable. A first-degree relative with a history of GDV, lean body mass index (BMI), deep or narrow thoracic conformation, stress, aggressive or fearful behavior, once-daily feeding, dry food and rapid food consumption, past splenic disease, and increased gastric ligament laxity are additional risk factors that have been reported.

Diagnosis

- Based on signalment, history, and clinical signs
- Radiographs distinguish simple gastric dilation from GDV

Treatment

Correcting hypovolemia is the primary goal of treatment, which is achieved by quickly replacing lost fluid with the use of one or more large-bore (16–18 gauge) IV catheters put into the cranial (jugular, cephalic) veins. Prompt initiation of fluid treatment using crystalloids at the shock rate (90 mL/kg/hr) is recommended. When these products are utilized, the rate of infusion of crystalloid fluid can be reduced by as much as 40%. In cases of severe shock, an animal may benefit from fluid treatment that combines crystalloids, colloids (e.g., hetastarch administered intravenously at a rate of 10–20 mL/kg), or hypertonic saline (e.g., 7% hypertonic saline solution with dextran 70 administered at a rate of 5 mL/kg over 15 min). During stabilization, flow-by oxygen must be supplied.

Stomach decompression and the proper administration of fluids are typically involved in the treatment of electrolyte and acid-base imbalances. Due to the potential risk of endotoxemia and GI translocation of bacteria, antibiotics (e.g., ampicillin at 25–50 mg/kg, IV, every 6–8 hours, and continued for 2-3 days following surgery) are routinely administered.

Cooperative gastric decompression is performed with fluid resuscitation. The initial attempts at decompression should be performed with an orogastric tube. Following sedation, it can be used with or without diazepam (0.1-0.2 mg/kg, slow IV) or hydromorphone (0.1-0.2 mg/kg, IV infusion, to effect) or fentanyl (2-5 mcg/kg, IV, once). Avoiding vasodilating medications (such as phenothiazines) is advised. A stomach tube that is marked and measured precisely from the incisors to the last rib is employed. The tube cannot go beyond this marking. The lubricated tube is inserted into the dog's mouth while it is sitting (occasionally held open with a cotton gauge, bandage, or tape). At the esophageal-gastric sphincter, non-compliance is usually present to some extent.

The tube may need to be gently manipulated and rotated counterclockwise in order to pass into the stomach, but caution must be exercised because the tube has the potential to pierce the esophagus. As soon as the tube reaches the stomach, gastric contents swiftly escape.

The insertion of a gastric tube does not eliminate the risk of volvulus. To slow down the rate of redilation with gas, the stomach should be lathered with warm water after the gas and contents have been released via the tube.

If an orogastric tube is difficult to pass, percutaneous gastrocentesis may be used to release extra stomach gas. A portion of the right abdominal wall (10 cm × 10 cm) is prepared aseptically from the caudal region to the final set of ribs. and ventral to the process of the transverse spine. Tympany should be indicated by percussion in the region, preventing inadvertent splenic puncture. The surgical correction of GDV occurs shortly after the initial stabilization.

Analgesia and IV fluid therapy are two instances of postoperative medical care. After surgery, food should be avoided for 48 hours. Antiemetic medications (maropitant at 1 mg/kg/day, SC; metoclopramide at 0.2-0.5 mg/kg, SC, or 1-2 mg/kg/day, constant-rate IV infusion) may be administered in cases of persistent vomiting.Owners of breeds where the risk of GDV infection is high should be informed about the disease's risk factors and symptoms, and they should seek veterinary care as soon as any clinical symptoms develop.

Traumatic-Reticulo-peritonitis (TRP)

The cattle and buffaloes ingested a sharp object (such as a nail or wire) that punctured the reticulum wall, resulting in reticulum wall inflammation in that area. Traumatic reticulo-peritonitis is the name given to this illness. Goats and sheep, for example, are picky feeders and have far lower disease rates than other ruminants.

Clinical signs

Reduction in feed intake, bruxism, tachycardia, decreased rumen motility, mild fever, poorly digested feces, arched back, erect hairs at the withers, tense expression, hesitancy to move, and a careful walk are the most common clinical symptoms. Animals can be made to grunt for diagnostic purposes by offering food, leading them down, or expressing pain signs (Fig. 23.2).

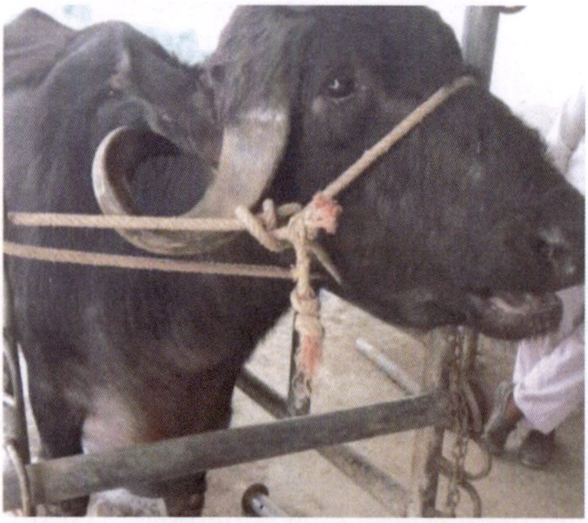

Fig. 23.2. A female Jaffarabadi buffalo with TRP is expressing signs of pain.

Diagnosis

- Clinical assessment
- Foreign body tests (such as the pole test, reticulum percussion with a hammer or mallet, or back grip) to elicit a grunt reaction
- Laboratory testing (such as peritoneal fluid D-dimer concentration or differential serum-to-peritoneal fluid glucose concentration)
- Radiography
- If any foreign materials are present, radiography makes them visible. Ultrasonography testing is necessary to locate and detect inflammatory reticular lesions.

Treatment

The first step in treating traumatic reticulo-peritonitis in cattle is to give them a rumen magnet (one magnet per animal, if the animal does not already have one). Magnets lessen stress by causing ferromagnetic foreign items to accumulate in the reticulum and rumen. The effectiveness of the rumen magnet depends on the position of the foreign body within the reticulum; foreign bodies that are upright or on the ventral aspect of the reticulum are easier to detect with a magnet than those that are either penetrating the reticulum or not in contact with it.

Antimicrobial medication (such as penicillin or broad-spectrum antibiotics; for example, tetracyclines at 10–20 mg/kg, IM, every 24 hours, ceftiofur at 1.1–2.2 mg/kg, and ampicillin at 4.4–11 mg/kg, IM, every 24 hours; or 22 mg/kg, SC, every 12 hours). Anti-inflammatory medications such as meloxicam (0.5–1.0 mg/kg, IM, every 24 hours), ketoprofen (3 mg/kg, IM, every 24 hours), and flunixin meglumine (2.2 mg/kg) are administered to relieve pain.

The optimum course of treatment for traumatic reticulo-peritonitis is rumen magnet and antibiotic therapy; laparo-rumenotomy is sometimes performed in optional situations if medicinal treatment is not successful.

References

Borakhatariya, D. and Gadara, A. (2017). Surgical management of choke through oesophagotomy in a buffalo: A case report. Indian Journal of Veterinary Sciences & Biotechnology, 12(3), 73–74.

Braun, U., Gerspach, C., Ohlerth, S., Warislohner, S. and Nuss, K. (2020). Aetiology, diagnosis, treatment and outcome of traumatic reticuloperitonitis in cattle, The Veterinary Journal, 255, 105424.

Cheng, K.J., McAllister, T.A., Popp, J.D., Hristov, A.N., Mir Z. and Shin H.T. (1998). A review of bloat in feedlot cattle. Journal of Animal Science, 76(1): 299–308.

Ducharme, N.G., Hackett, R.P., Ducharme, G.R. and Long, S. (1983). Surgical Treatment of Colic Results in 181 Horses. Veterinary Surgery, 12: 206-209.

Eggertsdottir, A.V. and Moe, L. (1995). A Retrospective Study of Conservative Treatment of Gastric Dilatation-Volvulus in the Dog. Acta Vet Scand, 36:175–184.

Guilford, W.G. and Strombeck, D.S. (1996). Acute gastritis. In: Guilford WG, Center SA, Strombeck DR, editors. Strombeck's small animal gastroenterology. ed 3. Saunders; Philadelphia.

Kumar V, Vadalia JV, Patel AM, Prasad A, Talekar SH and Patel PB (2016). Ultrasonographic, radiographic diagnosis and management of esophageal obstruction in Jaffarabadi buffaloes and Gir cattle. Buffalo Bulletin 35(4): 549-556.

Spielman, B.L. and Garvey, M.S. (1993). Hemorrhagic gastroenteritis in 15 dogs. J Am Anim Hosp Assoc, 29:341.

24

Gynaecological Emergency

Pratyush Kumar, Abhishek Kumar, Raju Kumar Dewry and Nancy Jasrotia

Key Points

- In dairy cows, anestrus is a prevalent reproductive condition.
- In dairy farm animals, infertility, pyometra, and repeat breeder cows are the main reproductive syndromes.

Introduction

Farm animals have been raised and chosen specifically for the production of meat and dairy over the years. The livestock business suffers significant financial losses as a result of farm animal infertility. If the open span is extended by one estrous cycle as a result of infertility, this explains the 20–25 day loss of output in addition to the expense of treatment, missed work, etc. Farm animals can become infertile for a variety of reasons, including nutritional deficiencies, physiological disorders, and viral infections. These factors can act alone or in concert.

Because of this, every case needs to be precisely evaluated and treated in accordance with the conditions identified during the examination. Infertility is caused by certain metabolites and nutritional variables, according to recent studies. The luteinizing hormone secretion frequency and dynamic follicle diameter decreased during the postpartum energy deficit, although the calving interval time rose. Animals that are infertile, subfertile, or sterile can be identified by careful examination of their health and management. Infertility is influenced by a variety of factors, including management, infectious agents, and nutrition. Mineral supplements, balanced feeding, and green fodder are examples of nutritional factors. Breeding plans, prompt oestrus identification, maternity care, postpartum care for moms, and immunization schedules for key diseases are examples of management facets. Genital tract infections can be caused by bacteria, viruses, protozoa, and fungi.

Infertility in cows

One of the main factors influencing a cow's lifetime performance is her fertility. Every 12 to 14 months, a calf needs to be produced for dairy cows. Farm animals can become infertile for a variety of reasons, including nutritional deficiencies, physiological disorders, and viral infections. These factors can act alone or in concert.

Both in terms of the expense of maintaining a cow and the missed revenue opportunity from having fewer calves available for sale, economic losses can be significant. If the next calving time is prolonged, there will be more losses, which will raise production costs and result in lighter calves that are weaned the following year.

It is feasible to identify infertile animals only through extensive management and health screening research. Mineral supplements, balanced diets, and the addition of green fodder can reduce nutritional concerns. Regular deworming and immunization schedules, breeding policies, prompt oestrus identification, postpartum care for animals, and care for pregnant animals are all examples of management-related factors. The following discusses a few of the infertility-related problems that are frequently seen in field settings.

Anestrus

The general term "anestrus" refers to the absence of estrus expression at the anticipated time. The ovaries are quiescent, inert, and devoid of functional corpus luteum (CL) during genuine anestrus. Malnutrition, lactational stress, seasonal stress, chronic wasting disease, senility, and other factors may be at blame for this.

Prepubertal anestrus

- undernutrition-related delayed puberty;
- abnormal reproductive system conditions, such as freemartins, hermaphrodites, segmental aplasia of the paramesonephric duct, and ovarian hypoplasia;
- and debilitating illnesses, including recurrent pneumonia, among others.

Postpartum anestrus

- physiological anestrus for two to three weeks following delivery;
- lactational stress; nutritional effects, such as imbalanced energy and micronutrient deficiencies;
- uterine diseases, such as retention of fetal membrane (RFM), metritis, pyometra, etc.;

- and chronic, crippling conditions, such as displaced abomasum, hardware disease, or leg injuries.

Post-service anestrus

- Pregnancy
- Pyometra
- Luteal cyst

Treatment of true anestrus

1. By using the right medication, such as fenbendazole or albendazole, for deworming.
2. Feed concentrate rations supplemented with a mineral mixture
3. Three days of intramuscular phosphorus injection (10 milliliters; tonophosphan)
4. Applying Lugol's iodine to the external os and gently massaging it three times on different days
5. Herbal heat-inducing medications, such as Prajana, Sajani, Janova, Fertikit, etc., can be utilized in cases where the aforementioned conventional treatments are ineffective. Oral Prajana HS 3 capsules every day for 2 days. Repeat after ten days if she doesn't come into heat.
6. Hormone treatment: The administration of comparable GnRH Receptal (Buserelin 20 mg) 5 ml I/M can be administered based on the reproductive organs' condition.
7. When there is quiet heat, inject any PGF2alpha analog while active CL is still present, and then perform double AI after 48–72 hours.

Management of Cystic Ovarian Degeneration (COD)

The term "ovarian cyst" refers to follicle-like ovarian formations with a diameter of 2.5 cm or more, which typically occur in the absence of the corpus luteum and last for 10 days or longer. These cysts cause abnormal reproductive function. The primary cause of COD is a deficiency in LH secretion during the pre-ovulatory phase.

Follic cyst clinical indicators include nymphomania, which is characterized by excessive and protracted oestrus signals and a short gap between two successive oestruses, excessive vulva enlargement, and more frequent and copious vaginal discharge than usual. Make an attempt to mount other cows and refuse to be mounted by them. Bull-like in its sexual behavior, the afflicted cow is commonly referred to as a "Buller". Anestrus, or the end of cyclic activity, is one of the clinical indicators of a luteal cyst.

Diagnosis

A clinical examination, combined with the patient's history and symptoms, is typically used to diagnose an ovarian cyst. A typical preovulatory follicle has a diameter of about 2.5 cm. Its palpable features, which include being a smooth, fluid-filled, structure with thin walls elevated above the ovary's surface, could be mistaken for a follicular cyst. See the variations in uterine palpation and associated symptoms for this. Transrectal ultrasound imaging has the potential to significantly increase diagnostic accuracy.

Treatment of Follicular Cysts

1. Manual rupture: Palpation of the rectum is used to manually rupture cystic formations. Manual rupture may be followed by ovarian hemorrhages and adhesions, which could worsen infertility. Therefore, it is best to discourage manual ruptures.
2. Gonadotrophin-releasing hormone (GnRH): Most cows that react to therapy with a GnRH analogue (Buserelin) enter the estrus 18 to 23 days following treatment. Receptal: 5 ml I/M (Buserelin).
3. Sequential GnRH and PGF2α therapy: When GnRH is administered, ovarian cysts that luteinize experience regression akin to that of healthy corpora lutea. The duration between starting GnRH medication and the onset of the first oestrus is shortened by 18 to 23 days due to PGF2α's luteolytic action. On the ninth day, PGF2α should be administered following GnRH medication.
4. Progesterone administration: a single dosage of 750–1000 mg of progesterone is used to treat follicular cysts, or 50–100 mg of progesterone (Duraprogen) I/M for 14 days.

Treatment for luteal cyst: Vetmate, 2 ml IM, or Lutalyse, 5 ml I/M, the PGF2α counterpart.

Repeat Breeder Cows

Known as a repeat breeder, a cow or buffalo with a normal or almost normal estrous cycle and estrus period has been artificially inseminated three or more times in a row to a fertile bull or with the semen of a fertile bull but has not succeeded in becoming pregnant. Repeat breeding syndrome is mostly caused by two factors: early embryonic mortality and fertilization failure.

Treatment

1. When environmental or external factors cause early embryonic death, appropriate care can help to correct this problem.

2. GnRH analogues stimulate ovulation during insemination. AI service providers need to be well qualified.
3. Early embryonic mortality is also brought on by subclinical uterine infections. Systemic or intrauterine antibiotic therapy is recommended for this. Pre-AI or post-AI antibiotic treatment is the most widely used course of action in practice.
4. The inseminated cow or buffalo should be kept in a cool area or shed for 15 days following insemination, since heat stress might cause embryonic death.
5. If an energy deficit is detected, intravenous 20% dextrose should be administered one to two hours prior to A.I.
6. 500 mg of progesterone (2 ml, duraprogen) should be injected intramuscularly after 5 days following insemination, and the procedure should be repeated on day 12.

Pyometra

Pus buildup in the uterus is accompanied by a chronic CL. The animal then enters an anestrus. When endometritis does not go away and an animal ovulates, causing CL to form, the condition may arise post-partum.

Clinical Signs:

In postpartum pyometra, the cervix does not remain too tight. So, some of the pus escapes when the cow lies down, urinates, or defecates.

- Not exhibit oestrum signs.
- Regarding peroral examination.
- The corpus luteum is present.
- The uterine wall is thicker than it was during pregnancy.
- The uterus stays swollen.
- There are no caruncles or fremitus; instead, the uterus is more "doughy," feeling like soft balls of wheat flour when fingers are forced into it.

Treatment

a) Analogs of PGF2α include Vetmate (2 ml I/M) and Lutalyse (5 ml I/M). Within five to seven days, these result in pus expulsion, cervical dilation, and regression of the corpus luteum. The symptoms of estrus suggest that the uterus needs to evacuate.
b) Parenteral antibiotics (ideally the penicillin group) should be given throughout the hormonal treatment to stop infection from spreading to

the oviducts as a result of uterine contraction. Additional antibacterials like fluoroquinolones and tetracyc1ines are also beneficial.

Care of newborn calves

1. Use your fingers to clear mucus out of your mouth and nose. Ribs and thoracic organ damage can occasionally result from overzealous chest compression. Even though the infant has a strong and healthy pulse and heartbeat, it is generally not expected that they will survive if resuscitation does not cause spontaneous respiration within two or three minutes. In certain instances, applying a mixture of corpropamide and crotethamide solutions to the tongue can increase respiratory activity.
2. The fetus will typically have mild respiratory and metabolic acidosis at the time of a normal birth; this can be treated fairly safely with a bolus intravenous injection of 50 to 100 ml (35 g in 400 ml of lukewarm water) of sodium bicarbonate at a dose rate of 1 to 2 mmol/kg.
3. The newborn's ability to regulate their body temperature: Try to have the delivery as soon as possible in a setting that is thermally neutral.
4. Preventing umbilical infections: If the chord hasn't broken, it should be cut with scissors around 2 inches from the umbilicus, and the stump should be disinfected with antiseptic. If the bleeding is not too severe, the navel cord should be left untied and allowed to drain. Apply the tincture of iodine to this stump. It is recommended to remove the ligation in a day or two.
5. Colostrum feeding: The first feeding should take place within the first two hours of the infant's life. If colostrum is unavailable, young animals of larger species should get subcutaneous injections of 200–500 ml of dam's blood serum, while smaller animals should receive injections of 20–100 ml.

References

Arthur's Veterinary Reproduction & Obstetrics. 8th edition. W.B. Saunders.

Hafez, E.S.E. and Hafez, B. eds., 2013. Reproduction in Farm Animals. John Wiley & Sons.

Kumar, P. 2009. Applied Veterinary Gynaecology and Obstetrics. 1st Edition, International Book Distributing Co. Noakes, D.E. and Parkinson, T.J. and England, G.C.W. 2001.

25

Obstetrical Emergency

Raju Kumar Dewry, Pratyush Kumar, Abhishek Kumar and Nancy Jasrotia

Key Points

- Dystocia, uterine prolapse, obstetrics, and torsion of the uterus are among the common obstetrical issues in dairy animals.
- These reproductive abnormalities cause dairy farmers to suffer significant financial losses.

Introduction

Every instance of obstetrical complications needs to be handled right away. Along with taking the case history, a general clinical assessment and examination should be performed. Dystocia is one of the various obstetrical problems that is more common in cattle.

The main obstetrical issues in dairy animals are listed here, along with management techniques for each animal.

1. Dystocia

Dystocia is a term for birth difficulties. It is a condition when the initial or second stages of parturition are noticeably extended, making it difficult or impossible for the mother to give birth to the child naturally.

Causes

- The most frequently impacted species is the bovine.
- Poor fetal appearance, posture, and position
- In primipara, as opposed to pleuripara, it is more prevalent.
- The primary cause of the heifers' delayed body and pelvic growth was inadequate nutrition during their growth.
- Little pelvis, an immature juvenile genital system, and insufficient strength to push out the fetus.

- Crossing a malnourished, underfed female that may be old enough to reproduce but whose body has grown much more slowly as a result of illness, parasites, or inadequate nutrition.
- Elevated feeding rates encourage the excessive accumulation of fat in the pelvic area, which makes parturition more difficult, particularly in heifers.

Overeating promotes the growth of a bigger fetus, which makes delivery difficult, especially in the final third of pregnancy.

- Dystocia can be caused by any infection or disease that affects the uterus and its contents during pregnancy.
- The prevalence is higher in heavier male calves, twin pregnancies, hydroamnion and fetal anasarca in cattle, and small litter sizes in multiparous species.
- Fetal malposition and uterine inertia are the main causes of dystocia in preterm pregnancies.
- The occurrence is increased by prolonged gestation leading to large fetuses, close overfeeding, close confinement, underfeeding, and premature breeding.

Clinical symptoms

- Having trouble giving birth.
- The calf's face or limbs sticking out of the vulva.
- The animal uses considerable force to try to deliver the calf but fails.

How to approach a case of Dystocia

Every dystocia case is a clinical issue that can be resolved with the right steps. Gathering a history from the owner or attendant, performing a targeted clinical examination, and doing a particular examination of the reproductive system are all necessary for the case to be managed successfully. Before making any corrections, it is important to distinguish between labor that is not fully formed and labor that has been interrupted. A thorough diagnosis of any defective fetal disposition should also be made.

Assistance required

- Having three assistants is ideal for the obstetrician/veterinarian. One person will handle the patient's head, and two will help deliver the fetus at the patient's back end and keep the cow from swinging her back end around while being examined and treated.
- If the cow chooses to lie down easily during delivery, her head should be secured low.

Management Methods

- It must be managed by a licensed veterinarian.
- Correcting the fetus's presentation, position, and posture
- It has been proposed that dairy heifers could be bred not by age but by weight or size.
- All animals should, if at all possible, be attentively observed during parturition so that, in the event that parturition is abnormal, quick assistance may be provided.
- At the time of service, the dam and sire should be clear of illnesses to help control the infections that can lead to uterine disease and fetal death.

Sedation

- Occasionally, an intramuscular injection of xylazine (5 mg/100 kg body weight) may be necessary for sedation prior to an internal examination for safety, particularly in cases involving unhandled and anxious heifers.
- Xylazine may make myometrial contractions stronger; however, this usually doesn't lead to any issues.
- When taken intramuscularly, clenbuterol at a dose of 300 mg for an average body weight of 200–250 kg will relax the uterus and lessen the force of uterine contractions caused by xylazine.

Epidural anesthesia

- It's only necessary during calving if the extreme strain on the mother makes handling processes like fetal repulsion extremely challenging.
- It is possible to stop frequent urination when handling.
- A typical cow should receive 5-7 milliliters of 2% lignocaine hydrochloride, as this helps to prevent straining and preserve the patient's capacity to stand.

Equipment

- Waterproof parturition gown and gumboots.
- Generally, protective sleeves and gloves are not worn unless an infection is suspected if the obstetrician's arms are sensitive to bovine vaginal fluids.
- Three colored nylon calving ropes with small wooden cylindrical handles;
- a sterile caesarean section surgery kit; a dystocia or foetotomy set.

Lubricant

For calving, there should be at least 750 cc of synthetic colloidal gel available since it is highly helpful. The conventional obstetrical lubricants are soap and water. You can also use liquid paraffin as a lubricant.

Warm water: 5-10 liters.

Drugs

- Tetanus anti-toxin, uterine pessaries, injectable antibiotics, calcium borogluconate, dextrose solutions, clenbuterol, or isoxsuprine.
- One should offer a systemic, broad-spectrum antibotic medication.

Conclusion

Dystocia cases are stressful situations that may affect the cow and the calf for the rest of their lives. Because they can result in cow injury or death, calf death, and veterinary expenses, they also cause farmers to suffer large financial losses. They may also make the cow less productive following the loss of a calf, which is bad for the wellbeing of the calf as well as the cow.

2. Uterine Prolapse

The evacuation of uterine mass through the vagina is known as uterine prolapse. It is a typical third-stage labor problem. Uterine prolapse is a common third-stage labor problem that is more common in cows and less common in ewes and other animals.

Major Causes

- Strong or violent tenesmus during or after childbirth.
- Placenta retention is near the uterine horn's ovarian pole.
- Excessive ease of movement in the pelvic and perineal areas.
- It is usually observed in cattle that are stabled or restricted, particularly in the winter.
- The fetus was extracted forcefully.
- A high intra-abdominal pressure level.
- The uterus contracts more slowly.
- Underweight heifers, an inadequate diet, and hypocalcemia can also result in uterine prolapse.
- Primary uterine inertia is a result of myometrial abnormalities from overstretching, impaired expression of prostaglandin or oxytocin receptors, and an increased risk of uterine prolapse. Additionally, hypocalcemia may cause the uterus to become atonic after labor

ends, delaying the cervix's and the uterus' involution. Second, there is a higher chance of prolapse if tenesmus persists beyond the second stage of labor. These circumstances include retained fetal membranes, laceration of the reproductive system, and the aftermath of a dystocia or forcible extraction of the fetus to address fetomaternal disproportion. Thirdly, extended periods of lying down, whether because of paralysis or hypocalcemia, are linked to an increased risk of prolapse. This may be because lying down causes an increase in intraabdominal pressure.

Clinical symptoms

- When the animal lies down, there is a slight protrusion of the vaginal mucous membrane through the vulval aperture.
- When standing, the prolapsed mass occasionally hangs down to the hock joint.
- Usually, the bulk is covered in blood clots, straw, dung, or dirt.
- Particularly in situations that are delayed (4-6 hours), the uterus is swollen and edematous.
- Normally, the cervix is located at the vulva.
- The non-gravid horn does not evert; instead, it is kept inside the prolapsed gravid horn's peritoneal surfaces.
- Animals may exhibit restlessness, nervousness, elevated heart rate, and stress.
- Internal bleeding resulting from a uterine vessel rupture, shock, intestine mass imprisonment, and demise.
- Pale mucous membranes, difficulty getting up, an expiratory grunt, and prostration accompanied by extreme sadness suggested significant problems.

Management Methods

Suggested first aid

- The animal with a prolapsed uterus should initially be kept apart from other animals. An epidural anesthetic is administered to minimize straining. The ability to stop defecating while the procedure is underway is another benefit. Giving a preparatory injection of calcium borogluconate to treat milk fever and reduce rumen tympany is a good idea.
- One way to handle the recurrence and backpressure in a recumbent animal is to elevate its hindquarters (by employing hip lifters or placing the animal on a bale of straw, for example).

- The prolapsed mass needs to be shielded from external sources of contamination of any kind.
- Until therapy, the bulk should be covered with clean, damp clothing.
- Managing this problem requires a competent veterinary doctor to carefully place the protruding uterine mass into the body and suture the vulval lips.
- It is recommended to administer tetanus toxoid, nonsteroidal anti-inflammatory medications, and suitable antibiotics as part of the postoperative care.

3. Torsion of Uterus

Torsion of the uterus, which occurs frequently in cows and buffaloes, is the twisting or turning of the gravid uterus on its long axis. It may be shown that pluriparous people have a higher occurrence than primiparous people.

Major Causes

- The disorder known as uterine torsion may be predisposed to frequent lying down and getting up.
- Pregnant animals kept in closed quarters without exercise are susceptible to uterine inertia and uterine torsion.
- Torsion may be more likely in cases of low fetal fluids, violent falling or rolling, and abrupt movements.
- Uterine torsion is favored by the pregnant uterus's lack of tone, which includes its small, non-gravid horn, loose walls, and absence of fluids.
- Because buffaloes have a propensity to wallow, a deep, capacious abdomen makes them more susceptible to uterine torsion.
- When pregnant animals are transported by train or road, their violent and erratic motions might induce anxiety and increase the risk of uterine torsion.

Clinical symptoms

- Observations may include pain in the abdomen, anorexia, constipation, absence of ruminations, restlessness or signs of colic, teeth grinding, treading, and tail switching.
- A shift in the dorsal commissure position.
- Vulval edema and tucked-up udder.

Prevention Method

- Pregnant animals should be handled with special caution and kept in separate housing. Pregnant animals should also not be transported.

- It is advisable to prevent pregnant animals from rolling, jumping, lying down frequently, and falling.
- It's best to stay away from animal fights and attacks.

Control Method

- Only a veterinary doctor with the necessary qualifications and skills should treat this problem.
- A veterinary doctor can assist with the rolling or rotation of the dam. In complex circumstances, a laparoscopy or cesarean section is advised.

4. Retained Fetal Membranes

One of the most prevalent ailments that animals have after giving birth is this one.

The primary reason of this is the fetal cotyledon's villi's inability to separate from the mother crypts of the caruncles and hold onto them for longer than usual. The situation is deemed pathological if the placenta is kept for more than 8–12 hours.

Major Causes

- Placental membrane retention may be the result of uterine infections during pregnancy.
- Inertia in the uterus brought on by hormonal imbalance, such as low oxytocin levels.
- Retained placenta is a result of vitamin A and iodine deficiency.
- Fetal membrane retraction may be brought on by an excess of cortisol and the hormone progesterone during the latter stages of pregnancy.
- The illnesses that lead to uterine atony or inertia increase the risk of retained fetal membranes.
- One of the main risk factors for retained placenta is close confinement and inactivity.

Clinical symptoms

- Even after the fetus is expelled, some of the fetal membranes remain attached to the vulva for up to 12 hours.
- Depression and anorexia could emerge.
- After the foetus is expelled, the placenta starts to macerate, which results in the development of a foul smell.

Control Method

- It must be removed manually by a licensed veterinary physician.
- The dangling fetal membranes should be shielded from dogs and other animals before the veterinarian arrives.
- To keep the protruding membranes from coming into contact with the hocks, tie them in a knot.
- It is possible to try manual removal between 24 to 48 hours of parturition.
- It is not recommended to remove the device manually after 48 hours because the cervix had closed.
- It is not advisable to manually remove the placenta from cows that have high body temperatures, vulvitis, or vaginitis.
- To avoid tetanus infection, a tetanus toxoid injection is advised following fetal membrane removal.

References

Dessie Abera (2017). Management of Dystocia Cases in the Cattle: A Review. Journal of Reproduction and Infertility 8 (1): 01-09.

Gordon, I.A.N. (1996). Controlled Reproduction in Cattle and Buffaloes. 1st ed. Wallingford: CAB International, 1: 202.

http://www.agritech.tnau.ac.in/expert_system/cattlebuffalo/Obstetrics%20and%20Gynecological%20conditions.html#:~:text=A%20lack%20of%20tone%20of,because%20of%20the%20wallowing%20habit.

Pradeep Kumar (2009). An approach to a case of Dystocia. In Applied veterinary gynaecology and obstetrics by, 1st Edition

26

Mammary Emergency

Anand Mohan

Key Points

- In diary animals, the health of the mammary gland (udder) is paramount.
- Any udder or teat disease state has a direct impact on milk output.
- Common udder/teet affections include: abscess, mammary gland hematomas, udder cleft dermatitis, udder edema, intramammary hemorrhage, teat damage, ulcerative mammillitis, udder dermatitis, and more.

Introduction

Mammary gland (udder) health is a crucial factor in animals used for production. The state of the udder determines the dairy industry's economics. The output of dairy animals is directly impacted by any udder ailment. Due to selection, breeding, genetic engineering, and animal management, animals under production pressure are more susceptible to a variety of diseases. More safety measures should be implemented in order to shield the udder from illness-causing factors. The many udder and teat affections and their therapeutic management are briefly discussed in this chapter.

1. *Mastitis*

In terms of monetary losses for dairy animals in India, mastitis is one of the main problems. Mastitis consumption not only results in financial losses but also presents a serious risk to public health that affects all of humanity. Food poisoning, brucellosis, streptococcal sore throat, and tuberculosis can all be contracted from eating raw (unpasteurized) milk.

Regardless of the cause, mastitis is an inflammation of the mammary gland's parenchyma that is defined by pathological alterations in the glandular tissue as well as a range of morphological and chemical changes in the milk. Both symptomatic and subclinical mastitis are possible. Clinical mastitis is characterized by breast gland edema, discomfort, swelling, and warmth upon probing. Subclinical mastitis is more harmful and difficult to identify visually through milk testing or by manual palpation.

2. *Etiology*

It has a variety of causes; if the barrier or defense mechanism fails to keep the mammary tissue safe, outside microorganisms may infiltrate the tissue. Mastitis is brought on by bacteria, viruses, fungi, and mycoplasma. The teat canal is the primary route of infection for the mammary gland. Environmental and contagious mastitis pathogens are the two main types of mastitis-causing microorganisms.

i) ***infectious mastitis pathogens:*** Infected cows' glands are typically the source of infectious pathogens. *Staphylococcus aureus and Streptococcus agalactiae* are the most prevalent.

ii) ***Environmental mastitis pathogens:*** Streptococcus uberis, Streptococcus dysgalactia, Arcanobacterium pyogenes, and coliforms (especially *E. coli, Enterobacter* sp., *Serratia* sp., and *Klebsiella* spp.) are the pathogens that cause environmental mastitis. These infections originate from the surroundings of the cow.

Diagnosis

When an udder is palpated, it may become painful, firm, and red when the condition is clinical mastitis. It is possible to see flakes, clots, or serous, bloody, and watery discharges in milk.

Strip Cup Test: This test uses an enamel plate that has been divided into four strips cups. The bottom of the plate is colored black to make it easier to see the milk flakes when the cups are tilted at an angle. The diagnosis of clinical mastitis can be made with this test.

Wisconsin Mastitis Test (WMT): A quick screening test conducted at the cow's side. When milk is treated with WMT reagent, a gel forms, suggesting that there are more inflammatory cells present and that mastitis may be developing.

The test for measuring the pH of milk is called the bromothymol blue test.

Haematology and serum biochemistry: Due to the impact of severe infection and toxemia, there may be noticeable alterations in the leukocyte count, packed cell volume, serum creatinine, and urea nitrogen concentration in cases with severe clinical mastitis.

Somatic cell counts: As the most widely used indicator of milk quality and udder health, a rise in somatic cell counts is the most notable subclinical abnormality of the milk.

Dairy Herd Improvement Associations employ automated electronic cell counting technology called Electronic Somatic Cell Counting. The expense of the Electronic Somatic Cell Count apparatus and the requirement for ongoing monitoring are the main drawbacks.

The California Mastitis Test (CMT) is the most affordable and accurate test that can be performed on cows to identify subclinical mastitis. Only cell count variations greater than 3,000,000 cells/ml are displayed by the CMT.

Handling

The animal's health and the type of mastitis it has are the determining factors in the treatment plan. Clinical mastitis is usually treated with medical intervention.

i) **Antibiotic therapy:** Antimicrobial sensitivity testing and culture are used to determine which antibiotic is best for a given mastitis pathogen.

Table 1: Categorization of antibiotics according to their pattern of distribution in udder tissue after parenteral and intramammary administration

Extent of antibiotics distribution	Parenteral route	Intramammary route
Antibiotics with good distribution	Quinolones, Sulfanilamide, Erythromycin, Oleandomycin, Tylosin, Spiramycin, Lincomycin, Clindamycin, Penathamate, Trimethoprim, Tiamulin	Quinolones, Nitrofurons, Sulfanilamide, Dapsone, Erythromycin, Oleandomycin, Tylosin, Spiramycin, Lincomycin, Clindamycin, Penathamate, Ampicillin, Amoxicillin, Hetacillin, Cephalexin, Trimethoprim, Novobiocin, Rifamycin
Antibiotics with limited distribution	Penicillin G, Cloxacillin, Ampicillin, Amoxicillin, Cephalosporins, Tetracycline, Novobiocin, Rifamycin, Fucidic acid	Penicillin G, Cloxacillin, Oxacillin, Cephoxazole, Cephalonium, Cephapirin, Cephacetril, Tetracycline
Antibiotics with poor distribution	Dihydrostreptomycin, Neomycin, Kanamycin, Aminocidine, Spectinomycin, Gentamycin, Polymyxin, Vancomycin	Bacitracin, Neomycin, Tyrotricin, Dihydrostreptomycin, Aminocidine, Gentamycin, Polymyxin

(*Source*: Gruet et al., 2001. Advanced Drug Delivery Reviews)

ii) **Oxytocin treatment:** Intramammary drug diffusion is frequently hindered by the accumulation of inflammatory debris in alveoli and lactiferous ducts. In cases of clinical mastitis, it has been suggested to fully empty the quarter by administering a parenteral oxytocin injection (10–20 IU IM) and then manually strip the afflicted quarters before infusion.

iii) **Supportive therapy:** In cattle with severe systemic disease, substantial volumes of isotonic crystalloid fluids should be administered intravenously. NSAIDs, such as Dipyrone and ketoprofen, are helpful in lessening the severity of clinical symptoms.

iv) **Dry cow therapy:** This involves administering intramural antibiotic therapy as soon as the last milking occurs during lactation (around 60 days).High concentrations of antimicrobial drugs in a slow-release basis are found in intraamammary infusions used in dry cow therapy, which helps to sustain therapeutic levels in the dry udder for extended periods of time. Cephalosporins and cloxacillin are commonly used for this purpose.

v) **Antioxidant treatment:** A diet deficient in numerous vitamins and micronutrients, including copper, selenium, vitamin A, D, and E, increases the risk of developing mastitis, a longer-lasting infection with more severe clinical symptoms. Biological systems can suffer greatly from the effects of free radicals. In order to eliminate intracellular infections, phagocytic granulocytes also go through respiratory bursts that create oxygen radicals. If these oxidative products are not removed, they may cause harm to healthy cells. By stabilizing these extremely reactive free radicals, antioxidants help to preserve the structural and functional integrity of cells. Vitamins A, C, and E, as well as some trace minerals like selenium, are typically involved in tissue defense systems against damage from free radicals.

Due to its extremely poor likelihood of recovery, treating subclinical mastitis during lactation is typically not advised.

Prevention

- Good milking techniques and hygiene of the bladder
- Handling and treating dry cows;
- Keeping the animal's surroundings clean;
- Checking on the condition of the udders

3. *Udder edema*

Cake, or urine edema, can have either a physiological or pathological cause. A few weeks before calving, physiological udder edema appears, and it is more noticeable in heifers getting ready for their first calf. Edema quickly disappears after calving and returns to normal in about a week. The length of time that pathological edema lasts and the degree to which it returns to normal depends on the illness. The reason of udder edema can occasionally be attributed to an increased intake of potassium and sodium. It could also happen in the event of hypoproteinemia. To conclude the case of edema, the udder must be evaluated physically and clinically, the milk must be evaluated to rule out mastitis, and disorders like udder abscess or hematoma must be ruled out.

Clinical signs

The floor of the udder and back compartment are typically where oedema is most noticeable.Cows with moderate to severe udder edema usually have varying degrees of ventral edema that extends from the fore udder toward the brisket. Ventral edema associated with bladder edema pits can be either mild and fluctuating or solid and pitting.

Treatment

When edema threatens to undermine the udder support framework, treatment is required. When a cow is on the verge of giving birth and exhibits severe udder oedema along with one or more teat leaks, treatment is also recommended.

- Diuretics, such as furosemide at 0.5 to 1.0 mg/kg BW, should be taken once daily for two to four days, then the dosage should be reduced.
- Reducing salt consumption ought to be taken into account.
- If there is no recovery, there may be an underlying reason (usually infectious origin), in which case treatment will be administered.

4. *Intramammary hemorrhage*

When there is severe udder edema or pendulous udders that have been injured by hind leg movement and awkward posture during recumbency, there is an intramammary hemorrhage. During parturition, bleeding into one or more glands is also commonly seen.

Indications

- Bloody milk needs to be adequately analyzed because blood is a great breeding substrate for germs and the likelihood of mastitis must be disregarded.
- Bloody milk contains blood from one or more quarters. It is red in color rather than pink. There are blood clots in the milk.

Treatment

Reducing the frequency of milking (usually to once a day) is the recommended treatment for intramammary hemorrhage. In the event that it doesn't resolve the problem in a few days, Adrenochrome (10 ml IM in large animals) might be given.It's critical to rule out coagulation abnormalities such as thrombocytopenia as probable reasons of the hemorrhage. Choosing the best course of action for hemorrhage can be difficult because iatrogenic problems can occur.

4. *Teat injury*

Animal teat injuries are caused by any physical harm to the teat (Fig. 26.1). Teat injuries are often caused by the finger or medial dewclaw of the injured cow's ipsilateral limb, or by a neighboring cow treading on the teat. Cows with pendulous udders are more likely to sustain injuries to the teat end. Teat injuries can also result from malfunctioning milking machines or from improper hand milking.

Indications

Mammary soft tissue swelling is most frequently observed near the distal teat. The skin could be hyperemic or injured. Any handling of the teat end irritates the cow.

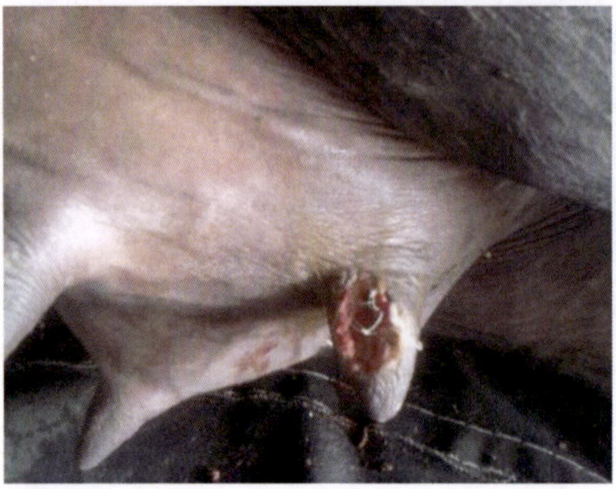

Fig. 26.1. Teat injury in a Murrah buffalo.

(*Source*: Kumar et al. (2014). Reconstruction of large teat fistula in buffaloes. Buffalo Bulletin 33(1): 19-21)

Treatment

After treating acute teat-end injuries, any management problems (overcrowding, lack of bedding, problems with the milking equipment, etc.) should be addressed.The best therapies for acute teat injuries involve minimizing further stress to the teat and symptomatic anti-inflammatory therapy. Using a sterile teat cannula, milk twice a day is recommended for optimal outcomes. After complete milkout, the teat end is dipped as usual, and a second dip takes ten minutes to complete.

5. *Abscess*

Abscesses can appear as hard, warm swellings that are either easily separated from or indistinguishable from gland parenchyma, and they can form anywhere in the mammary tissue. The swelling may be hard when palpated (Fig. 26.2). The milk from the affected quarter is usually normal as long as the abscesses are well-encapsulated. Endogenous abscesses can be the consequence of mastitis with abscessation caused by Arcanobacterium pyogenes.

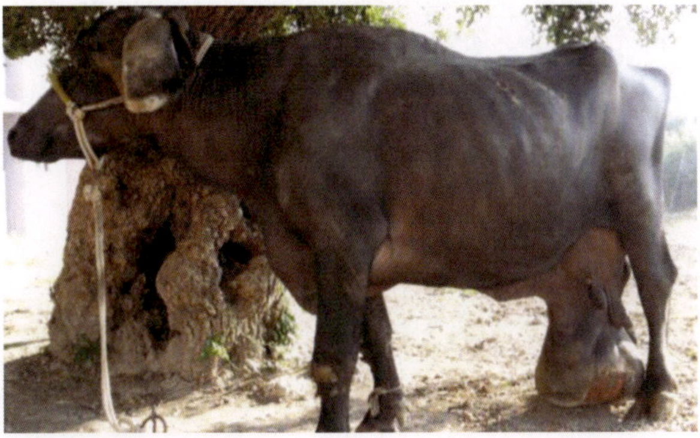

Fig. 26.2. Chronic udder abscess in a Jaffarabadi buffalo.

Diagnosis

Physical symptoms are typically sufficient for diagnosis. For more research, aspiration or ultrasonography may be employed.

Treatment

The best course of action is a conservative one that involves waiting for the abscesses to naturally rupture and drain in two to eight weeks as an open wound. Aspirating is advised prior to draining.After natural or surgical drainage, the abscess chamber should be cleansed once a day with diluted antiseptics or saline, and the drainage hole should remain open. Depending on the situation, supplements with antibiotics, antipyretics, antihistaminics, and vitamin B complex may be given.

6. *Ulcerative mammillitis*

The main causes of ulcerative mammillitis in dairy cows are Bovine Herpesvirus (BHV) () II and IV, which produce ulcerative conditions of the teat and udder skin (. The most frequent outcome of ulcerative mammillitis is decreased milk output, which is followed by bacterial mastitis. The majority of afflicted cows are those in their first lactation; however, exposed cows of any age might also get sick.

Clinical manifestations range from minor ulcerations to extensive edema plaques. Vesicles have a tendency to burst fast, producing a painful, ulcerated area that is covered in a dark-colored scab (Fig. 26.3). Often, the scabs rip up and bleed, especially when you try to milk them. In general, teats hurt. It may take several weeks for severe lesions to heal.

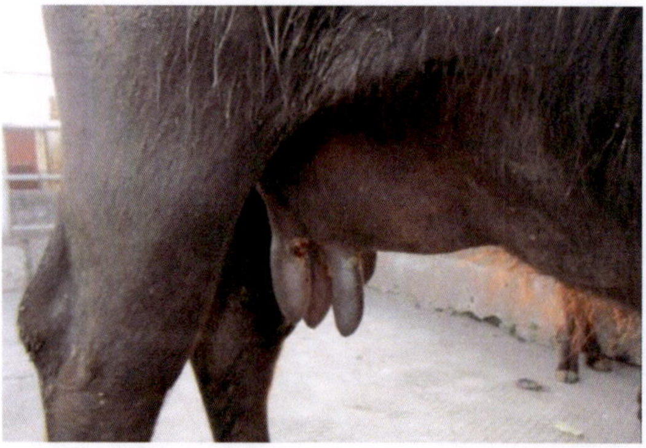

Fig. 26.3. Ulcerative mammilitis in a cross-breed Murrah buffalo.

Diagnosis

Diagnosis isbased on clinical signs and for confirmation, virus isolation from sample taken from early stage lesions is done.

Treatment

- Since the virus is the etiology, there is no proven treatment available; supportive care is the only recommendation.
- To inactivate the virus, food dips enhanced with emollients and iodophor can be utilized. Utilize different equipment for milking.
- Using single-use towels, wash and dry the teats.
- Wearing clean gloves during milking is recommended to stop the disease from spreading to animals that are vulnerable.
- Using a milk siphon to drain the milk ensures less manipulation of the mammary tissue, which further minimizes tissue damage.
- It is possible to supplement with broad range antibiotics, antipyretics, anti-inflammatory drugs, and vitamin B complex.

7. *Udder cleft dermatitis*

The most common term for udder cleft dermatitis, or udder sore, is a foul-smelling, wet dermatitic lesion. A risk factor is pressure necrosis of the udder skin, which is typically caused by periparturient udder engorgement or edema. The ventral midline portion of the udder or the groin area are where it most frequently occurs.

Indications

The unpleasant stench associated with wet dermatitis is similar to that of septic metritis or a retained placenta. In the worst situations, large skin portions (10 to 30 cm in length) may peel off. Scratches, matted hair, and necrotic skin are all present. Warm weather can cause myiasis to develop. Some first-calf heifers can develop lameness due to severe groin infections.

Handling

The best way to treat udder cleft dermatitis is with a topical wound spray that contains trypsin, castor oil, and balsam of Peru.Give furosemide intramuscularly (IM) at a dose of 1 mg/kg BW. The healing process may take months to finish in untreated circumstances. If the inguinal lesions are significantly limiting movement, surgical debridement could speed up the healing process.

8. *Udder dermatitis*

The irritation of the udder skin is called udder dermatitis. It could be brought on by physical irritation (such sunburn, frostbite, and pressure necrosis), chemical irritation (like irritants in bedding like hydrated lime, ammonia from urine), or fungal and bacterial involvement.

Signs

The indications differ according to the cause of the lesions. Chemical and physical teat skin dermatitis are characterized by extreme erythema, edema, and pain. Vesicles may be observed in cases of severe chemical irritation. The hair could seem a little matted and heavy with serum.

Treatment

- Aloe or lanolin products can be used to treat chemical dermatitis after the udder has been carefully cleaned in warm water and the offending ingredient has been removed from the skin.
- The best way to treat dermatitis with a physical cause is to relieve the symptoms while avoiding reintroducing the specific physical cause into the body.
- If photosensitization is the underlying cause, cows with sunburns need to be kept inside or in the shade; further exposure to sunlight needs to be avoided.
- Protecting against more injury and carefully and precisely debriding necrotic tissue are the only possibly viable therapies for frostbite.Cows with decubital sores or pressure necrosis should be given soft bedding.
- Hair on the udder is clipped, povidone iodine scrub solutions are gently used, water is rinsed, and the animal is dried. Next, antibiotics such as penicillin at 22,000 IU/kg body weight, OD IM for 5 to 7 days are administered in addition to local therapy to treat bacterial infections.

- Fungal lesions can be treated by clipping the udder's hair and then topically applying clotrimazole or miconazole ointments once or twice a day.

9. *Mammary gland hematomas*

Udder hemorrhatomas can cause severe blood loss because blood can build up subcutaneously. Soft tissue swells cranial to the udder are more common in lactating dairy cattle. The swelling may be mild, firm, or variable, depending on the quantity of blood accumulation. Palpation usually reveals it to be cool and painless.

Identification

The absence of fever, gradual anemia, and varying swelling in the vicinity of the udder are typically enough to establish the diagnosis. Aspiration under sterile conditions is necessary to differentiate a hemoatoma from an abscess or seroma when the diagnosis is unclear.Ultrasound might be performed to confirm.

Treatment

Mammary gland hematomas must be carefully managed with rest and careful observation of the animal every 12 to 24 hours. A coagulation test and complete blood counts (CBCs) should be performed to rule out bleeding problems. NSAIDs ought to be avoided while there is active bleeding.

Cutting into a bladder hematoma should not be done since it will make the bleeding worse. In stable udders, hematomas gradually reabsorb. Surgical debridement of naturally draining hematomas is not recommended, unless in chronic situations.

References

A text book of the diseases of cattle, sheep, pigs, goats and horses by Radostits O. M., Gay C. C., Blood D. C. and Hinchcliff K.W., 10th edition, Saunders Publication.

Gruet P, Maincent P, Berthelot X and Kaltsatos V, 2001. Bovine mastitis and intramammary drug delivery: review and perspectives. Advanced Drug Delivery Reviews. 50(3):245-59.

Kumar V, Ahmad RA, Amarpal, Pathak R, Hoque M (2014). Reconstruction of large teat fistula in buffaloes. Buffalo Bulletin 33(1): 19-21.

Textbook of Clinical Veterinary Medicine by MC Sharma, Mahesh Kumar and RD Sharma (2009). Directorate of Information and Publications of Agriculture, ICAR.

27

Musculoskeletal Emergency

Mamta Mishra

Key Points

- The main objective of managing open fractures is to neutralize further damage to the surrounding tissue while executing prompt, stable osteosynthesis and immobilization.
- Discomfort management should be considered because musculoskeletal diseases can cause severe discomfort.

Degenerative Myopathies

It is a degenerative disease of the musculature. Endocrine imbalances (hyperadrenocorticism, hypothyroidism, and hyperthyroidism), hypokalemia in cats, ischemic myonecrosis in recumbent cattle, post-exercise rhabdomyolysis, chemical agents, poisonous plants, and drug-induced degenerative conditions are some of the possible associations with it.

Clinical signs

Gait abnormalities, tachycardia, polypnea, high temperature, pain, and myoglobinuria (azoturia), etc.

Necropsy findings

Affected skeleton muscle has a white, waxy, and swollen appearance (fish flesh). Also, it shows pale and dry discoloration, white streaks, calcification, and intramuscular oedema.

Diagnosis

Based on the patient's medical history and symptoms. During the acute phase, measurements of lactate dehydrogenase, aspartate amino transferase, and creatinine phosphokinase are raised in the serum. It is advised to measure serum creatinine, selenium, and glutathione peroxidase levels further. There are varying degrees of hyponatremia, hypochloremia, and hyperkalemia seen.

Treatment

It is advised to inject or subcutaneously provide vitamin E and sodium selenite at doses of 10–40 IU/kg of food and 0.1–0.15 mg/kg, respectively.

Horses with exertional rhabdomyolysis should be treated with phenylbutazone at 2.0–4.4 mg/kg BW b.i.d., aspirin at 10–20 mg/kg BW orally spaced 48 hours apart, and injectable ketoprofen at 2.2 mg/kg BW b.i.d. Through a stomach tube, 2-4 mg/kg BW of diluted normal saline are administered as diethylene sodium. For clinical evaluation, xylazine hydrochloride may be given intramuscularly (IM) at 0.1–1.1 mg/kg BW/day in horses and 0.05–0.15 mg/kg BW/day in cattle.

Degenerative joint disease

Degenerative joint disease (DJD) is a kind of osteoarthritis or arthritis brought on by the gradual deterioration of one or more joints' articular cartilage. All conditions that cause inflammation in the joints are collectively referred to as arthritis.

Clinical signs

Osteoarthritis symptoms include lameness, joint edema, muscular atrophy, and thickening and scarring of the joint membrane. Joint movement may produce a grating sound when sufficient damage is done.

Diagnosis

The diagnosis will be made using clinical symptoms and radiography (X-rays will show increased fluid within the joint, soft-tissue swelling around the joint, the formation of bony outgrowths, hardening and thickening of bone beneath the cartilage, and occasionally a restricted joint space).

Treatment

The goal of treatment is symptomatic, and lifestyle modifications including losing weight and exercising under supervision are frequently advised.

Ibuprofen 5–15 mg/kg body weight PO TID and aspirin 25–50 mg/kg body weight PO TID are recommended for dogs. Carprofen at 2.2 mg/kg bdy wt. PO BID, indomethacin at 1-1.5 mg/kg bdy wt. PO TID, and PO TID are recommended for pain treatment.

Oral prednisolone tablets at a dose of 2 mg/kg body weight every day for a few days, then 1 mg/kg body weight as maintenance has been recommended in certain cases beforehand. In addition, joint supplements such as glucosamine glycan and chondroitin sulphate are recommended at 1 tab PO BID if the body weight is 30-35 kg and TID if the body weight is 35 kg or above. Supplements containing multiple vitamins and minerals are advised.

Laminitis

Horses and ruminants with sensitive foot laminae are susceptible to laminitis, an inflammatory disease.

Etiology

Other reasons include colic (anterior enteritis, big colon volvulus), acute postparturient metritis (retained fetal membranes), excessive carbohydrate ingestion (grain overload), cold water, and enterocolitis. Equine metabolic syndrome-related laminitis is most prevalent in overweight horses and ponies, and it is frequently made worse by rich pasture grazing. Acute ingestion of lush pasture may generate a combination of metabolic syndrome and sepsis-related laminitis, which is comparable to grain overload.

Any time a horse bears too much weight on one limb for an extended period of time due to an inability to utilize the other limb (such as following orthopedic surgeries, radial nerve paralysis, or an infected joint or tendon sheath), it can result in supporting limb laminitis.

Clinical findings

1. The animal will be depressed, anorectic, and will stand unwillingly with fluctuating lameness in the early stages of laminitis. Resistance is encountered throughout any exercise, and the standard posture is modified in an effort to lessen the weight supported by the injured foot (Fig. 27.1).
2. The sole is more sensitive and the digital arteries are beating faster.
3. The horse will stand with its forelimbs extended if they are the only parts hurt. The horse takes on a stooping, low stride when forced to walk.
4. The animal will appear "camped out," with the forelimbs positioned more frontally and the rear limbs positioned more caudally, if all four limbs are wounded. Every foot is lifted and then promptly placed down.

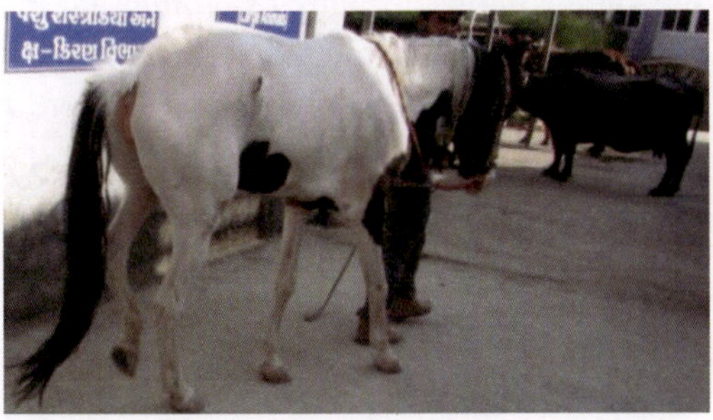

Fig. 27.1. Laminitis in a Marwari mare.

Necropsy findings

The secondary epidermal laminae totally disintegrate in extreme circumstances. Abscessation in necrotic laminae is conceivable. Rotate or sink ventrally, depending on the distal phalanx. Osteomyelitis or severe distal phalanx resorption may happen in extreme cases.

Diagnosis

It is recommended to obtain a patient's medical history, do a complete blood count (CBC), radiograph the limb in question, and assess clinical signs and symptoms.

Treatment

A laxative or purgative (mineral oil at 3–4 L) is advised in case of grain overload. It is recommended to use fluid treatment. Phenylbutazone can be given intravenously at a dose of 8.8 mg/kg body weight. After that, it can be taken 4.4 mg/kg body weight BID for a few days, and then 2.2 mg/kg body weight BID. BID: 10 mg/kg body weight of aspirin, 0.1–1 g/kg body weight of DMSO, and 1.1 mg/kg body weight of flunixine meglumine every 24 hours. Horses can get acetylpromazine at a dosage of 0.044 mg/kg bdy with water for four to five days. It is not advised to use corticosteroids.

Fracture

The normal structure and position of bones are often disrupted when a fracture occurs. Fracture reduction is the process of placing broken bones back where they belong anatomically. First aid can be used to treat distal transverse fractures, distal luxations, and septic arthritis, as general suggestions. It is possible to refer proximal luxations, oblique fractures, comminuted fractures, and proximal fractures (humeral, femoral, tibial, and radial).

Clinical signs

A broken limb manifests itself in a variety of ways, including swelling, immobility, whimpering, pain at the site of injury, limping or holding up the damaged leg or limbs, soft tissue bruises, abnormal angulation of the broken limb, and more.

Diagnosis

- X-rays of the injured location or sites; anesthetic may be administered to enhance comfort during this procedure.
- A CT scan can be helpful, particularly in cases with fractures to the jaw, skull, and spine.

Treatment and Management

Without requiring surgery, closed fractures can be reduced by carefully tractioning and managing external fragments. Using casts, splints, and bandages to immobilize a limb is known as external coaptation (EC) (coapt = approximation) (Fig. 27.2). This can be used as the main method of fixing, temporarily after surgery to offer additional support, or until permanent stabilization is accomplished. Open reduction necessitates surgical intervention.

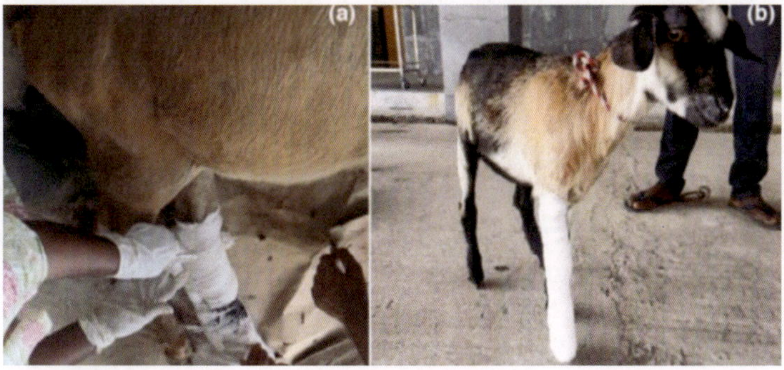

Fig. 27.2. External coaptation for immobilization of fractured limbs in a Purnea cattle (a) and a goat (b).

Closed Fracture Reduction

- Stabilize the animal by administering shock therapy and stabilizing its respiration, airway, and cardiovascular system.
- To gently and deliberately overcome muscle contraction, use traction, countertraction, and manipulation.
- When a patient has a distal limb fracture, they should be in a dorsal recumbency position and have their wounded limb suspended from a pole or ceiling hook. To increase the amount of countertraction and gravitational pull, they should raise the limb attachment and physically drag the animal off the table.

After reduction is complete, install the suitable external fixation or coaptation.

Limbs distal to the elbow or stifle joint can be momentarily immobilized using a Robert Jones bandage or modified Robert Jones. To achieve consistent compression of the distal limb, it depends on a secondary layer that is incredibly thick, like cast padding or cotton, and is then forcibly squeezed. Tightening the outer protective layer has little chance of impairing blood flow because of the thick cushioning.

Casts can be used as definitive therapy, as an adjuvant following surgical stabilization, or to provide temporary support for fractures or joint injuries while surgery is being performed. Casts encircle the limb entirely. Fiberglass cast or plaster of Paris is the material of choice since it produces a cast that is both lightweight and extremely stiff. The distal limb is wrapped in a modified Robert Jones bandage, with the exception of the outer layer of protection. The bandage should have an even, wrinkle-free surface and not be overly thick to keep the cast from coming loose. To initiate the setting process, the fiberglass casting tape is submerged in water while wearing gloves; any extra water is disposed off.

After that, the tape is unrolled over the softly padded bandage from distal to proximal. It is imperative to prevent folds, creases, or indentations in the cast as they may lead to pressure necrosis underneath. Additionally, at the ends of the bandage, the casting material must not come into contact with skin. The limb is covered with two to three layers of casting tape, overlapped by thirty to fifty percent. To stop excessive soiling, an external protective layer can be applied once the cast has hardened. Splints only shield the affected limb on one side. There are prefabricated splints (spoon and lateral splints) made of aluminum or plastic. When a distal femur fracture cannot be wrapped, the Schroeder-Thomas (ST) splint is utilized to support the fracture. A sturdy lateral support splint that curves over the shoulder or pelvis is combined with a soft, cushioned bandage to provide a Spica splint that maintains the forelimb or the pelvic limb in extension. Forelimb use of this splint is most common following reduction of elbow luxation. Avoid extended immobilization to prevent joint damage and muscle contracture. Other than that, nervine supplements, calcium, and NSAIDs are recommended.

References

Anderson DE., Jean SG (1996) External Skeletal Fixation in Ruminants, Veterinary Clinics of North America: Food Animal Practice, 12(1), 117-152.

Ferguson JG. (1982). Management and repair of bovine fractures, Compendium on Continuing Education for Practicing Veterinarians.

Lundvall RL. (1960) Fractures of the long bones in large animals, J Am Vet Med Assoc

Reichel EC. (1956). Treatment of fractures of the long bones in large animals, J Am Vet Med Asso.

Singh J., Singh S., and Tyagi, RPS (2019). The Musculoskeletal system: Ruminant Surgery: A Textbook of the Surgical Diseases of Cattle, Buffaloes, Camels, Sheep and Goats [CBS Publishers & Distributors]:423-527

Slatter DH. (2003). Musculoskeletal system: Textbook of Small Animal Surgery [Saunders], Vol 2: 1774-2285

28

Respiratory Emergency

Anand Mohan

Key Points

- Dogs exhibit respiratory distress symptoms more frequently than cats.
- Respiratory distress might have overt or covert clinical symptoms.
- The thorax and belly move paradoxically in cases of severe respiratory distress.
- Immediate intubation is the first step in managing a respiratory emergency: opening the airway.

Introduction

The telltale symptoms of "oxygen hunger" include tachypnea, stretched head and neck, abducted elbows, flare of the nares, cyanosis, open-mouth breathing, anxiety, and inability to lie down or relax. It is more usual for dogs than cats to exhibit symptoms of respiratory distress. Tachypnea and conspicuous breathing motions when in a sternal recumbency position are the only indications of respiratory dysfunction in cats, who often mask the severity of their illness. Despite their seeming stability, these patients are often extremely vulnerable and can rapidly decompensate when under stress.

There are five breathing patterns commonly seen in animals for respiratory distress.

1. Upper airway blockage manifests as loud breathing and inspiratory stridor. In extreme situations, inspiration causes the abdomen to pull inward, leading to paradoxical movement. The animal could exhibit anxiety and cyanosis symptoms. Possible causes include foreign body, nasopharyngeal polyp, pharyngeal/laryngeal edema, mass, bleeding, laryngeal paralysis, collapse of the trachea, and brachycephalic airway syndrome. The physician should be ready to conduct an emergency tracheostomy or to sedate and intubate the patient if intubation is not possible. Anxiety is frequently treated with a modest dose of acepromazine (30–50 ug/kg IV or IM), butorphanol (0.2 mg/kg IV), and

midazolam (0.25 mg/kg IV). If the body temperature rises, cooling with a fan and IV fluids can be necessary.

2. Rapid, shallow breathing and hushed heartbeats are signs of pleural space disease. Abdominal movements are paradoxical in severe situations. To stabilize the patient, an emergency thoracocentesis ought to be carried out. If fluid is recovered, the diagnosis might be made by microscopic cytology analysis. Should air be drawn out, note the volume and repeat thoracocentesis in 20 to 30 minutes if required. If air or fluid cannot be removed from the pleural space adequately, a thoracic drain may need to be inserted and possibly continuous suction may be necessary.
3. A symptom of a small airway disease like feline asthma, chronic bronchitis, or chronic obstructive pulmonary disease (COPD) is prolonged expiration with an expiratory push. In an emergency, cats with asthma are treated with corticosteroids (0.2 mg/kg dexamethasone IV or prednisolone sodium succinate at 2-4 mg/kg IV) and bronchodilators (0.01 mg/kg IM Terbutaline). Options for inhalation therapy include cromolyn, albuterol, terbutalane, and fluticasone.
4. Parenchymal diseases, such as pneumonia, pulmonary neoplasia, infiltrative illness, pulmonary contusions, and cardiogenic and non-cardiogenic pulmonary edema, are characterized by labored inspiration and expiration. Wheezes, crackles, and harsh lung sounds can all be heard during auscultation. The symptoms of congestive heart failure include tachycardia and a heart murmur. If the physician believes that congestive heart failure is the root cause of the patient's respiratory discomfort, they should give intravenous furosemide (2 mg/kg IV q 12 h with severe disease).
5. Primary lung illness is not usually the cause of tachypnea. Anemia, shock, pain, agitation, anxiety, fever, and metabolic acidosis must be ruled out as causes of tachypnea if the lung sounds are auscultatory.

General steps for management of respiratory emergencies

When dealing with a respiratory emergency, the first thing to do is intubate the patient right away to open their airway. Before beginning intubation, the airway should be free of secretions, foreign objects, and other impediments if it is not patent. The animal should then be ventilated with 100% oxygen at a rate of 20–30 breaths per minute. If tracheal intubation is not possible due to an upper airway obstruction, an emergency tracheostomy ought to be carried out. Choosing whether to anesthetize or sedate an animal in respiratory distress is a decision that clinicians frequently struggle with. If possible, supplemental oxygen should be given via a face mask or "flow by" while the patency of the airway is being assessed.

Ketamine (5 mg/kg), Midazolam (0.25 mg/kg) IV, or etomadate (0.5 - 2.0 mg/kg IV) can be utilized to induce fast induction with minimum cardiac depression if there is no improvement and an airway assessment and intubation are necessary. Although thiopental (5–10 mg/kg IV) and propofol (3–8 mg/kg IV) have been related to more severe cardiopulmonary depression in critically ill patients, they may still be utilized.

The combination of sedation and rapid intubation enables the medical professional to manage the animal's airway and, ideally, prevent intubation following cardiacCritical patients can receive oxygen by a variety of techniques, each with pros and cons of their own.

"Flow-by" oxygen (flow rates ranging from 3 to 15 L/min) is easy, affordable, and practical to give to critically ill patients during the initial assessment. Although face masks can also provide oxygen, some animals will resist them and become even more agitated when they are used.

For cats or dogs in such severe respiratory distress that even light handling puts them at risk of decompensation, an oxygen cage can be helpful. The patient can "chill out" in the oxygen cage's oxygen-rich atmosphere while the doctor keeps an eye on their breathing pattern.

Oxygen cages have the drawbacks of being expensive and requiring a lot of oxygen to fill. Moreover, it is simple for animals housed in an oxygen-tight cage to overheat. Although they are more costly, temperature and humidity-controlled cages are safer. Only temporary care should be provided with an oxygen cage in the absence of these attributes.

For animals in respiratory distress, nasal oxygen (flow rates of 50-100 ml/kg) is an inexpensive and efficient oxygen supplement. It makes it possible to provide the patient oxygen continuously while radiography, ultrasounds, physical examinations, and other treatments are being carried out. Before a nasal oxygen catheter is inserted, the nose is given a few drops of lidocaine or proparicaine. A feeding tube or lubricated 5–10 F red rubber catheter is inserted into the ventral meatus up to the level of the mandibular ramus (nasopharyngeal) or medial cathus (nasal). Pushing the planum nasale dorsally and directing the tube ventromedially facilitates easier passage of the tube in dogs. The tube can be fastened just above the naris, over the nose bridge, or on the lateral aspect of the face with suture, staples, or super glue. It is frequently necessary to use an Elizabethan collar to prevent the patient from pulling out the tube. Nasal oxygen is contraindicated in patients with thrombocytopenia.

Following the administration of supplementary oxygen, it is imperative to perform a comprehensive physical examination and closely observe the patient's breathing pattern.

There are some respiratory emergencies in which immediate attention required is listed below-

- Laryngeal obstruction
- Tracheal and tracheobronchial obstructions
- Tracheal collapse
- Laryngeal paralysis
- Aspiration pneumonia
- Pleural effusion

The best way to treat the aforementioned disorders is through surgery; for instance, obstructions in the larynx, trachea, or trachea-bronchial junction needed to be treated right away. The main focus should be on intubating the patient to maintain the patency of their airway. Later, the blockage will be surgically removed.

Both laryngeal paralysis and pleural effusion typically worsen over time and are most frequently linked to other medical conditions. In this case, there is enough time to diagnose the illness and start treating it appropriately. In field conditions, aspiration pneumonia is the most frequent case encountered. Although aspiration pneumonia has a poor prognosis, treatment for the condition began with large dosages of broad-spectrum antibiotics along with supportive therapy based on the patient's clinical symptoms.

The illness problems listed below, which are briefly discussed below, can result in respiratory crises.

1. Pulmonary edema

Pulmonary edema arises from the accumulation of fluid in the pulmonary interstitial alveolar spaces, and airways.

Causes

- Increased pulmonary vasculature hydrostatic pressure,
- Decreased pulmonary oncotic pressure,
- Obstruction of lymphatic drainage, or
- Increased capillary permeability.
- Decreased plasma oncotic pressure with albumin <1.5 g/dl
- Pulmonary thromboembolic disease,

- Severe upper airway obstruction (noncardiogenic pulmonary oedema),
- Seizures, and head trauma

Diagnosis

- Clinical signs of respiratory distress
- Presence of crackles on thoracic auscultation
- Cyanosis and fulminant blood-tinged frothy oedema fluid may be present in the mouth and nostrils.
- Thoracic radiographs and an echocardiogram

Therapeutic management

- Supplemental oxygen should be administered along with furosemide (4–8 mg/kg IV, IM). Fluids should be stopped if fluid excess is detected as a result of intravenous fluid therapy.
- Thoracic radiographs and an echocardiography should be performed once the patient has been stabilized initially in order to evaluate the cardiac side, pulmonary vascular size, and cardiac contractility.
- It is important for the clinician to ascertain whether increased permeability, hypoalbuminemia, pulmonary vascular overload, or volume overload are secondary causes of congestive heart failure causing pulmonary edema.
- Vasodilators, diuretics, oxygen, and occasionally positive inotropes are used to treat heart failure.

2. Chronic Obstructive Pulmonary Disease (COPD)

A chronic inflammatory disease affecting the respiratory system, COPD damages the lungs. This is a slowly progressing, irreversible condition. "Chronic bronchitis" is another name for this illness.

Reasons

- Exposure to inhaled irritants may cause long-term inflammation of the respiratory tract.
- A Bubbly Image

Clinical conclusions

- Chronic coughing in its early stages, or coughing that lasts more than a month.
- The cough is typically harsh or "dry," and gagging is frequent following a cough.

- Breathing difficulties and frequently a diminished tolerance to exercise
- The animal may start to wheeze as it exhales and start breathing noisily.
- Due to a shortage of oxygen, the gums may eventually take on a blue tint.

Diagnosis

- Heart rate is often normal or lower than normal with COPD, and a prominent sinus arrhythmia is frequently present.
- History.
- Auscultation reveals "crackles" (harsh crackling or popping noises).
- To rule out parasitic infections like lungworm or heartworm, a CBC, biochemistry profile, and certain blood or fecal tests may be advised.
- Radiology of the torso.
- Cytology using tracheal lavage and/or bronchoscopy.

Therapeutic management

- Cough suppressants;
- Bronchodilators (to widen the airways and facilitate secretion clearance);
- Antibiotics (in the event that a subsequent bacterial infection is suspected);
- Corticosteroids (to reduce inflammation and reduce coughing).
- Refraining from irritating substances like smoke and airborne allergens

3. Bronchospasms

The ailment known as bronchospasms, or bronchial asthma, is more common in some dog breeds, including pugs, because of the way their airways are shaped.

Causes

- Pollens
- Grasses
- Chemicals such as cleaners, shampoos, soaps, fragrance, sprays/ powders
- Smoke (cigarette or fireplace)
- Mold
- Dust mites
- Air pollution

Clinical signs

- Dry coughing (dry, hacking)
- Superficial breathing, as the airways are constructed and the animal will have difficulties breathing
- Wheezing
- Lethargy
- Purple gums and tongue, but only in severe cases
- Respiratory distress (difficulty breathing, shortness of breath, wheezing, dyspnea)
- Open-mouth breathing
- Exercise intolerance
- Lack of appetite
- Weight loss

Diagnosis

- Clinical signs and history
- Chest x-rays.
- Bronchial lavage.

Therapeutic management

- Untreatable, but medicine may help control
- To avoid severe episodes, the steroids should be taken on a regular basis. Severe asthma episodes may also require oxygen therapy.
- It's crucial to identify the triggers that cause your pet's asthma attacks and keep them away from them.
- Antihistamines or bronchodilators, which will help clear the airways and allow the animal to breathe.

4. Pulmonary thromboembolism

The blockage of one or more pulmonary arteries by a thrombus or embolus that originates elsewhere in the body is known as pulmonary thromboembolism.

Causes

- Hyperadrenocorticism,
- Disseminated intravascular coagulation (DIC),
- Catheterization of blood vessels,
- Bacterial endocarditis,

- Protein-losing nephropathy or enteropathy,
- Hyper viscosity syndromes,
- Heat-induced illness,
- Pancreatitis, Diabetes mellitus,
- Inflammatory bowel disease, and
- Immune-mediated hemolytic anemia.

Clinical signs

- A sudden onset of tachypnea, tachycardia, and cyanosis.
- if the embolism is big, the patient might not react well to extra oxygen delivery.
- Sudden, severe breathing difficulties.
- Continuous panting;
- Restlessness, anxiety, and pacing.
- An elevated respiratory rate greater than 40 beats per minute (bpm).
- Breathing with your mouth open.
- Blue-tinged gums (which, if left untreated, could result in death).
- Breathing through the neck; sitting up and spreading the front legs and elbows (as in an English bulldog position); and using the abdomen to improve breathing.
- Unexpected demise.

Diagnosis

- Radiographic findings.
- Clinical indicators of respiratory distress.
- A lung perfusion scan or angiography is necessary for a definitive diagnosis.
- Echocardiography can reveal tricuspid regurgitation, pulmonary hypertension, enlargement of the right heart, and indications of underlying cardiac illness, potentially with atria clots.

Therapeutic management

The management should include treatment and elimination of the underlying disease.

- Thrombolytic treatment, oxygen supplementation, and cardiovascular shock therapy
- Give heparin for short-term therapy.

- Tissue plasminogen activator, streptokinase, or urokinase are examples of thrombolytic treatment.
- It could be necessary to use low molecular weight heparin or warfarin for an extended period of time in order to stop additional thromboembolic episodes.

Bibliography

A text book of the diseases of cattle, sheep, pigs, goats and horses by Rodostits O. M., Gay C. C., Blood D. C. and Hinchcliff K.W., 10th edition, Saunders Publication.

MSD Veterinary manual. Available at https://www.msdvetmanual.com/emergency-medicine-and-critical-care/evaluation-and-initial-treatment-of-small-animal-emergency-patients/initial-triage-and-resuscitation-of-small-animal-emergency-patients.

Singe J Plunkett (2000). Emergency procedures for the small animal veterinarian. 2nd edition. WB Saunders.

Cefotaxim sodium at 5-7 mg/kgb.wt

Norfloxacin @ 10-15 mg/kgb.wt

Cephalosporin @ 5-7 mg/kgb.wt

Sulphonamide + Trimethoprim at 80-100 mg/kgb.wt

Note: To control side effects of drugs, i.e, crystal urea and calculi formation especially in canine urinary alkalizer like ALKASOL SYRUP, and NEERI TAB/ SYRUP with adlibitum drinking water is advised or Dextrose 5% at 20-50 mg/kg b.wt i.v, to increase urine outflow.

B. Urinary sedative

C. Antispasmodics

Inj Dicyclomine (spasmovet®) at 10 ml/large animal and 1-2 ml/small animal.

Catheterization is to be done to clear the retained urine.

Nephritis: Inflammation of kidney cells.

1. Glomeruli nephritis (glomerulus cell)
2. Interstitial nephritis (interstitial cell)
3. Pyelonephritis nephritis (parenchymal and pelvic cell)

Causes

- Bacterial (C. renale, E.coli, Leptospira spp. etc)
- Virus (Adenovirus, canine hepatitis virus, etc.)
- Parasites (Dictophyma renale, Dirofilaria imitis)
- Chemical
- Drugs like aminoglycosides.

Symptoms

Anorexia or polyphagia, polydipsia, polyuria, oliguria, anuria, dysuria, pyouria, hematuria, proteinuria, and edema on a dependent part of the body may present.

Treatment

- Judicious use of antimicrobial therapy for sufficient duration
- Diuretics
- Steroidal anti-inflammatory in tapering dose.
- An intravenous isotonic dextrose saline for prevention of dehydration.
- Animals should provide salt salt-free diet and adequate drinking water.

Urolithiasis

Anywhere in the urinary system, there is a deposit of crystals. The symptoms of urolithiasis include distention of the bladder or, in more severe cases, rupture of the bladder (Fig. 29.1), frequent attempts to urinate that are unsuccessful, and urine retention. It affects castrated males more frequently than females.

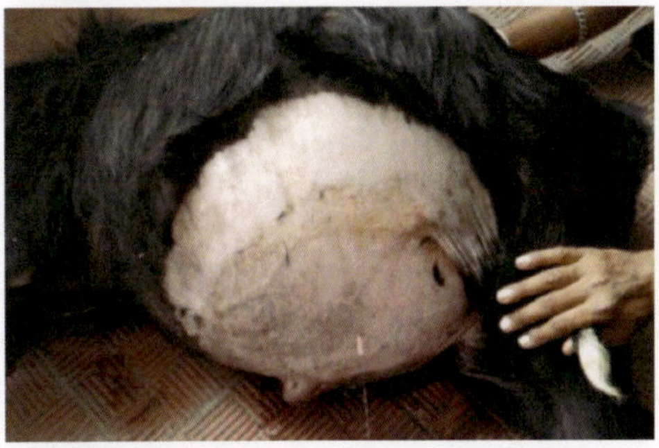

Fig. 29.1. Free-flowing urine through an 18-G needle in a male buffalo calf with urinary obstruction.

Table 29.1. Species-wise common site of urinary obstruction.

Sr. no	Species	Common site of urolithiasis
1	Bovine	Sigmoid flexure of penis
2	Caprine	Urethral process at tip of the penis
3	Equine	Ischeal arch
4	Canine	Proximal to the os-penis and neck of urinary bladder
5	Feline	Urethra

Causes

- Decrease intake of water and more consumption of hard water (chalky water).
- Mineral imbalance in feed, especially with reference to calcium and phosphorus.
- Chronic inflammatory condition of the urinary tract.
- Retention of urine and altered pH of urine.
- Vitamin A deficiency.

Symptoms

- Severe tummy ache accompanied by kicking.
- Excessive straining to get a pee.
- Pee dribbling or hematuria or dysuria.
- An enlarged urethra and bladder.

- In the severe stage, uremia and anorexia occur after the bladder bursts and all discomfort signs go away.

Treatment

- For ram/buck, calculi formation in the urethral process can be treated with a surgical nick; calculi formation in the urethral route necessitates a surgical correction called TUBECYSTOTOMY or URETHROTOMY.
- An ample supply of drinking water must be provided.
- Cystone tablet@1-2tabs TID for 30 days in ram/buck and canine.
- The following stone neutralizer medications should be used:
  a) Ammonium chloride at 200–400 mg/animal daily in 3–4 split doses for 11 days (for herbivores urinary acidifier medication).
  b) Sodium acid phosphate at 200–300 mg/cat or dog, PO for eight hours. Time intervals.
- Depending on the pH of the urine, urinary alkalizer drugs like Alkasol® syrup, etc., may be used for carnivores.

Diuretics

Use cautious when using them as they are not very helpful in urinary system illnesses. These aid in the elimination of waste and toxic products of metabolism in ascites and edema, among other toxicities. Take furosemides (Lasix®, Redima®, etc.) at doses of 2-6 mg/kg IM or IV.

Notes

Anuria: complete cessation of urine flow.

Oliguria: reduction of production and flow of daily quantity of urine.

Polyuria: increase of production and flow of daily quantity of urine.

Glycosuria: presence of glucose in urine.

Ketonuria: presence of ketone bodies in urine.

Pyouria: presence of pus cells in urine.

Proteinuria: presence of protein (albumin) in urine.

Difference between hemoglobinuria and hematuria is listed below

Sl. No.	Parameters/ Criteria	Haemoglobinuria	Haematuria
1	Urine	Presence of Hb in urine	Presence of blood in urine
2	Lysis of RBC	Yes	No
3	Urine colour	Deep red to brown (coffee) colour	Red colour

30

Metabolic Emergencies

Komal and Richa Arora

Key Points

- Electrolyte Imbalance: Regularly monitor and rectify imbalances in potassium, sodium, and other electrolytes dependent on the individual situation. Prompt management requires early detection of metabolic emergencies.
- Fluid Management: To restore intravascular volume and prevent dehydration in many metabolic emergencies, adequate fluid replacement is essential.
- Continuous monitoring of vital signs, laboratory values, and clinical status is essential for evaluating the efficacy of interventions and making necessary modifications.

Introduction

A class of disorders known as "metabolic emergencies" affect metabolism and physiology abnormally in both congenital and acquired forms. Among these ailments are endocrine disorders, thyrotoxicosis, inborn metabolic inefficiencies, and illnesses linked to electrolyte imbalances. Hypercalcemia, hyponatremia, hypoglycemia, hyperglycemia, and diabetic ketoacidosis, as well as hyperuricemia, hyperuremia, and hypercreatininemia due to renal failure, lactic acidosis, hyperammoniemia, and adrenal failure, are metabolic emergencies that pose a life-threatening risk.

Hypercalcemia

An excessive rise in the blood level of calcium is known as hypercalcemia. Bones that are robust and healthy require calcium. Calcium is essential for numerous physiological processes, including blood coagulation, neuromuscular, cardiovascular, endocrine, and immunological activities. The parathyroid glands interact with vitamin D to monitor and regulate calcium levels, which allow calcium to be released from the bones, kidneys, and stomach and into the bloodstream. Hypercalcemia is a serious condition that can lead to several medical emergencies, such as cardiac dysrhythmia, renal failure, mineralization of the kidneys, and other soft tissues.

Elevated calcium levels have been linked to a number of severe conditions as secondary symptoms, such as cancer, Addison's disease, hypervitaminosis D, acute and chronic kidney failure, parathyroid gland tumors, granulomatous inflammation, and bone illnesses related to osteolysis. Bone fractures are more common in dogs.

Diagnosis

- Serum biochemistry profile along with an ionized calcium test.
- Complete blood count.
- Parathyroid hormone test (PTH).
- Physical examination with peripheral lymph nodespalpation.
- ACTH stimulation test.
- Urine sample to see the kidney damage.

Mild hypercalcemia may not require treatment; calcium levels may progressively return to normal, and the doctor will monitor the kidneys' health. In case the calcium levels rise more or fail to return to normal on their own, doctors might suggest further testing.

Hyponatremia

The most common disruption to the body's fluid and electrolyte balance observed in clinical settings is hyponatraemia, characterized by a drop in plasma sodium content of less than 140 mEq/L. Since the plasma Na^+ concentration mostly determines plasma osmolality, hyponatraemia leads to hypoosmolality. Hypoosmolality usually indicates a kidney defect or excess water in the body because of increased collecting tubule permeability, insufficient ADH secretion, and adrenal insufficiency because the renal system is engaged in water excretion. In addition to neurological symptoms, hyponatremia can produce twitching of the muscles, vomiting, low blood pressure, appetite loss, and energy loss. The three distinct kinds of hyponatremia—hypovolemic, hypervolemic, and euvolemic—are distinguished by the reasons behind the imbalance between sodium and water in the body.

Diagnosis

- Metabolic panel
- Osmolality blood test
- Osmolality urine test
- Sodium urine test

Dialysis is a treatment option for severe cases of hyponatremia, along with the use of diuretics, or medications that retain sodium, and an intravenous infusion of a sodium solution.

Hyperuricemia

A rise in the blood level of uric acid, a nucleotide degradation product, is known as hyperuricemia. This happens when the body can't get rid of enough uric acid or produces too much of it. A high uric acid level causes crystals to develop in the kidney or around the joints. Joint crystals create arthritis, which results in inflammation and pain around the joints, and kidney stones cause fever, nausea, vomiting, stomach pain, and bad odors in the urine.

Diagnosis of hyperuricemia

- Blood test
- Urine test

Allopurinol is commonly used as a first-line urate-lowering medication (ULT) for treatment. Nonsteroidal anti-inflammatory medicines (NSAIDs), such as ibuprofen, can also be prescribed by doctors.

Hyperuremia

A clinical condition called hyperuremia is defined by elevated blood urea levels. Kidney disease is the cause of this disorder, which is linked to electrolyte, fluid, metabolic, and hormone imbalances. More cases of this illness are observed in chronic renal disease, particularly in its last stages. Numerous tissues are either directly or indirectly impacted by urea. Hyperuricemia may impact the central nervous system, resulting in cephalalgia, myalgia, exhaustion, wasting, convulsions, and unconsciousness.

Diagnosis

- Urine test
- GFR or creatinine clearance test
- Blood test

For treatment, dialysis is suggested.

Hypercreatininemia

A clinical disease known as hypercreatininemia is characterized by an elevation of creatinine in the blood. Creatinine is a waste product produced by muscles that is normally removed by the kidney. Elevations in blood creatinine may not be dangerous in and of themselves, but they may indicate a number of illnesses, including chronic kidney disease (CKD). Vomiting, nausea, elevated blood pressure, cramping in the muscles, altered urination patterns, dehydration, and fluid retention are all symptoms of this illness. Kidney stones, glomerulonephritis, and infections are the causes of it. Creatinine levels are also elevated in patients with diabetes and heart disease.

Diagnosis

- Blood test
- Urine test

Treatment includes the use of antibiotics.

Hyperammonemia

It's a metabolic disorder marked by elevated ammonia (a nitrogen-containing molecule) levels. Ammonia is a waste product that the intestine produces when breaking down proteins. The liver processes it, and the urea cycle eventually gets rid of it. Headache, nausea, vomiting, lack of appetite, seizures, and coma are symptoms of this illness. Ammonia causes the process of hyperventilation to accelerate, which also results in respiratory alkalosis. A malfunction in the urea cycle is typically the cause of hyperammonemia. Other metabolic disorders, such as organic acidurias, liver disease, and problems with fatty acid oxidation, are also linked to this illness.

Diagnosis

- Measuring plasma ammonia
- Plasma and urine amino acid profiles

Treatment includes protein intake discontinuation, treatment with nitrogen scavengers, and glucose.

Adrenal failure

The adrenal glands' hormone production is necessary for the body to function properly. Insufficient hormone production by the adrenal glands causes this disease. It can be primary, meaning that adrenal gland injury results in insufficient synthesis of cortisol and aldosterone, or secondary, meaning that the pituitary gland produces insufficient amounts of ACTH (adrenocorticotropin). Muscle weakness, hypoglycemia, low blood pressure, joint discomfort, nausea, vomiting, diarrhea, and loss of appetite are all linked to this illness. These illnesses can be brought on by medication side effects, pituitary tumors, autoimmune diseases, and hereditary problems.

Diagnosis

- Blood tests (potassium, sodium and pH blood tests)
- Insulin-induced hypoglycemia test
- ACTH stimulation tests

Treatment

- Injection of hydrocortisone sodium or hydrocortisone potassium succinate.
- IV saline solution into your vein in your arm or hand (intravenously).
- Hydrocortisone injection.

Lactic Acidosis

Lactic acid is typically created during normal physiological processes and is eliminated by the liver and kidney. When these organs are compromised, lactic acidosis results. A type of metabolic illness known as lactic acidosis develops when the body begins to produce more lactate as a result of tissues having less oxygen available to them, which eventually raises the blood level of lactic acid. Jaundice, respiratory problems, muscle soreness, decreased appetite, diarrhea, exhaustion, a fast heartbeat, and headaches are all linked to lactic acidosis. Heart failure, diabetic mellitus, hypovolemic shock, and liver and renal disorders are the main causes of lactic acidosis.

Diagnosis

- Blood tests

Treatment

- By treating the root cause.
- By increasing oxygen availability to the tissues
- By giving IV fluids.

Diabetes

It is a metabolic illness that causes the body's ability to process blood sugar to be impaired, which eventually results in hyperglycemia, or elevated blood glucose levels. There are two varieties of diabetes: Type-1 and Type-2. An autoimmune disease known as type 1 occurs when immune cells target pancreatic cells, impairing the pancreas' ability to generate the hormone insulin, which is necessary for the breakdown of blood sugar. When the body's insulin receptors fail to react, Type 2 diabetes develops. Because insulin is the hormone that uses sugar for energy, hyperglycemia can occur in both types.

Diabetes results in a number of health problems, including weight loss, exhaustion, thirst, high blood pressure, frequent urination, impaired eyesight (diabetic retinopathy), kidney damage (diabetic nephropathy), and ketoacidosis. High blood sugar levels harm the retinal blood vessels in diabetic retinopathy, causing the blood vessels to enlarge and cause visual loss. Without insulin, the body cannot digest glucose in ketoacidosis; as a result, the liver continuously generates glucose to fuel the body, which accumulates in the bloodstream. When there was insufficient glucose available, the body switched to breaking down fat, which resulted in the production of ketone bodies and their accumulation in the blood.

Ketone bodies and glucose are excreted in the urine, where the kidneys must remove them with a large amount of water, which causes dehydration and eventually ketoacidosis.

Diagnosis of Diabetes

- Urine analysis
- Blood test
- Oral glucose tolerance test
- Hemoglobin A1C test

Treatment

- Oral insulin therapy
- Physical activity
- Implementation of diabetic diet

Hypoglycemia

This illness is characterized by a low blood glucose level of 70 mg/dl. Hunger, perspiration, exhaustion, weakness, tremor, convulsions, unconsciousness, and a fast heartbeat are among the symptoms. This illness is typically brought on by prescription side effects, kidney issues, fasting, increased physical activity, drug-induced hepatitis, insulin consumption, and pancreatic tumors.

Diagnosis

- Blood test

Treatment includes supplementation of carbohydrate and glucose.

Jaundice

Hyperbilirubinemia, another name for this metabolic condition, is characterized by a yellow discoloration of the body tissues brought on by an abnormal build-up of bilirubin, either from excessive production or from poor elimination. Bilirubin comes in two varieties: unconjugated or indirect (insoluble in water) and conjugated or direct (soluble in water). Following the heme's breakdown in the macrophage, bilirubin is produced, conjugated by glucuronic acid in the liver, and then eliminated through bile into the stool.There are three varieties that can occur: hepatocellular, obstructive, and pre-hepatic (hemolytic). Unconjugated bilirubin levels are higher in the prehepatic stage, conjugated and unconjugated bilirubin levels are higher in the hepatic stage, and excretion is impaired in the posthepatic stage. Fever, stomach ache, skin discoloration, and dark urine and feces are among the symptoms.

Diagnosis

- Urine test
- Physical examination
- Complete blood count
- Van Der Bergh test (Direct or indirect)
- Hay's test
- Fouchet test
- Ehrlich test

Blood transfusions, corticosteroid medicine, and diuretics are all part of the treatment.

References

Abboud, B., Sargi, Z., Akkam, M., & Sleilaty, F. (2002). Risk factors for postthyroidectomy hypocalcemia. Journal of the American College of Surgeons, 195(4): 456-461.

Bilous, R., Donnelly, R., & Idris, I. (2021). Handbook of diabetes. John Wiley & Sons.

Fargo, M. V., Grogan, S. P., & Saguil, A. (2017). Evaluation of jaundice in adults. American family physician, 95(3): 164-168.

Husebye, E. S., Pearce, S. H., Krone, N. P., & Kämpe, O. (2021). Adrenal insufficiency. The Lancet, 397(10274): 613-629.

Qian, Q. (2019). Hypernatremia. Clinical Journal of the American Society of Nephrology: CJASN, 14(3): 432.

Roglic, G. (2016). WHO Global report on diabetes: A summary. International Journal of Noncommunicable Diseases, 1(1): 3-8.

Sahay, M., & Sahay, R. (2014). Hyponatremia: A practical approach. Indian journal of endocrinology and metabolism, 18(6): 760.

Zagzag, J., Hu, M. I., Fisher, S. B., & Perrier, N. D. (2018). Hypercalcemia and cancer: Differential diagnosis and treatment. CA: a cancer journal for clinicians, 68(5): 377-386.

III Poisoning

31

Drug Poisoning

Diptimayee Sahoo

Key Points

- Drug poisonings can be acute or chronic and result in the development of clinical signs and symptoms that may lead to animal disability or death, as well as extreme physiological and/or psychological changes.
- Drugs are substances that are used to prevent, treat, diagnose, and relive disease conditions by changing the physiology and/or psychology of the individual.
- Certain veterinary drugs have a specific antidote to counteract poisoning cases, while other veterinary drugs do not, and supportive therapy is required to counter these poisonings.
- Over-the-counter (OTC) medications, which are defined as human drugs or nutritional supplements that are available without a prescription, have potential risks for use in animals due to their increased toxicity.

Introduction

Many veterinary medications, which are used to treat both animals and birds, have the potential to poison the species to whom they are provided. These medications' toxic effects are mostly caused by giving them to the wrong species, at the wrong doses, or in the wrong combinations of medications. Certain medication poisonings can be identified due to patient individuality and eccentricities. As a result, there are many cases of these poisonings. This chapter discusses the poisoning caused by frequently and carelessly used veterinary medications, such as the toxicity of antibiotics and antibacterials, the toxicity of antiparasitic drugs, the toxicology of analgesics, the toxicity of cough treatments, the toxicity of the digestive system, the toxicity of vitamins, and the toxicity of topical preparations.

Poisoning situations are frequently very challenging to diagnose. As a result, specifics regarding clinical, pathological, and circumstantial evidence are helpful in diagnosing a condition.

Key points for treatment of poisoning

1. ***Removal of unabsorbed poison***

a) Skin- wash the skin with cold water (don't use hot water). Avoid rubbing of the affected part or area.

b) Gastrointestinal tract-

- Gastric lavage using water or a neutralizing agent.
- In the event that stomach lavage is not available, two table spoons of table salt dissolved in warm water may be used as emetics.
- As a cathartic, one to two tea spoonfuls of sodium sulfate may be used. It should only be administered following gastric lavage.
- Only after gastric lavage should activated charcoal be administered, as it is an effective absorbent for both organic and inorganic substances.

2. ***Removal of absorbed poison***

a) By parenterally administering a 5-to 10% glucose solution or water (not saline) during kidney diuresis.

b) Inhaling clean air.

c) Intestinal Tract: Cathartics and sodium sulfate may be utilized.

3. ***Symptomatic and supportive treatment***

a) Preserving a clean airway by clearing obstacles

b) Stimulant-induced respiratory depression control.

c) Shock abatement: shielding against the cold, replenishing lost electrolyte and water, and oxygen therapy

d) Control seizures: administer barbiturates intravenously (IV); if this is not feasible, administer orally.

e) Infection control: Antibiotics can be used to treat secondary infections such skin vesicles, urinary tract infections, and bronchopheumonia.

Name of Drugs	Signs of poisoning	Treatment	Commonly affected animal spp.
1) Antibacterial and antibiotics toxicity			
I) Sulfonamides and Sulfonamide combinations	a) **Hypersensitivity reactions:** include urticaria, angioedema, anaphylaxis, skin rashes, drug fever, polyarthritis, hemolytic anemia, acute drug shock with collapse and death b) **Acute toxicity:** Salivation vomition diarrhea, polypnoea, weakness, ataxia, blindness and convulsion c) **Chronic toxicity**: • **Bone marrow depression**: Leads to aplastic anemia, granulocytopenia, and thrombocytopenia • **Renal toxicity:** Crystalluria, hematuria, albuminuria, obstruction of renal tubules and ureter and oliguria • **Hypoprothrombinemia:** Leads to prolonged bleeding and clotting time in poultry • **Keratoconjuctivitis sicca (KCS):** Occurs in dogs after prolonged treatment with sulfonamides • **Neurotoxicity:** Peripheral neuritis and myelin degeneration in the spinal cord and peripheral nerves (in chicken and cattle) • **Inhibition of carbonic anhydrase enzyme:** Leads to acidosis, production of thin or absence of eggshells in poultry as well as reduced egg production • **Hepatic necrosis:** Mostly seen in dogs • **Other symptoms of chronic toxicity :** hepatitis and icterus, photosensitization, stomatitis, conjunctivitis, iatrogenic hypothyroidism and goiter	• Discontinuation of the use of drug • IV fluid administration in dehydrated and crystalluria patients • Adrenalin and antihistamine administration in hypersensitivity reactions • Alkalization of urine using bicarbonates • Vit K1 administration in coagulopathy syndrome	Dog, cat, poultry, cattle

II) Tetracyclines	**a) GI upsets:** anorexia, abdominal pain, diarrhea, nausea and vomition **a) Effect on bone/teeth:** yellowish then brownish discoloration in teeth and bones and impaired healing processes in fractured bones, **a) Hepatotoxicity:** fatty infiltration of liver and jaundice **b) Nephrotoxicity:** acute tubular nephrosis in animals **c) Hypersensitivity reactions:** rare and includes urticaria, skin rashes, pruritus and exfoliative dermatitis	• Supportive and symptomatic treatment	Cattle, dog
III) Penicillins	**(a) Hypersensitivity reactions:** Vary from mild and transitory skin reactions to fatal anaphylactic shock (bronchospasm, complete airway obstruction and death). Acute allergic reactions in dog included labored breathing, salivation, shivering, vomition, urticaria and pharyngitis whereas in cattle included labored breathing, salivation, cutaneous edema of head and perineal region **b) GI disturbances:** Includes nausea, vomition, anorexia and diarrhea **c) Platelet dysfunction** **d) Neurotoxicity:** Seen as ataxia in dogs **(e) Cation toxicity:** Aggravates congestive heart failure	• Parenteral administration of adrenaline • IV fluid therapy • Maintainance of airway	Cattle, dog
IV) Aminoglycosides (Gentamycin, tobramycin, amikacin, kanamycin, neomycin, streptomycin)	**a) Nephrotoxicity:** proteinuria, crystalluria and renal failure **b) Ototoxicity:** nystagmus, incoordination, head tilt ataxia, loss of righting reflex in animals **(c) Neuromuscular blockade:** muscular weakness, apnoea, respiratory arrest	• Hydration of patient • Use of diuretics • IV administration of calcium salts or neostigmine in case of neuromuscular blockade	Cat, Dog
I) Fluroquinolones	**a) GI disturbances:** Includes nausea, vomition, anorexia, abdominal pain and diarrhea **a) Nephrotoxicity:** Crystalluria in dog **a) Effect on bone/teeth:** lameness and pain in growing animal because of degenerative lesions in the cartilage of weight bearing joints	• Hydration of patient • IV Fluid therapy • Use of diuretics	Dog, horse

(2) Antiparasitic drug toxicity			
I) Macrocyclic lactones (avermectins and Ivermectin)	**Clinical signs:** anorexia, salivation, dullness, reduced water intake and abdominal pain, hypermetria, shivering, mydriasis, ataxia, bilateral blindness, tremors and incoordination of gait, abnormal posture during recumbency and death	• Aggressive fluid therapy • Supportive treatment-liver extract with vitamin B complex, theophylline, chlorpheniramine maleate, diazepam and dexamethasone	Cattle, dog, horse, cats
II) Benzimidazoles	**a) GI upsets:** Anorexia, abdominal pain **b) Embryotoxicity and terratogenicity:** administration of drug during first trimester of pregnancy results in these severe effects	• Supportive treatment-liver extract with vitamin B complex • Hepatoprotectants	Cattle, dog
(3) Analgesic toxicity			
I. Acetaminophen (Syn. Paracetamol)	Anorexia, vomiting, salivation, apathy, dyspnoea, facial edema, recumbency, bleeding tendencies, icterus, hypothermia, acute keratoconjunctivitis sicca in dogs	• Fluid therapy Use of specific antidote, Acetylcysteine or *N*-acetylcysteine or NAC Hepatoprotectants Vitamin C administration Activated charcoal (in case of ingestion of high dose of drug)	Dog, cat
II. Non-steroidal anti-inflammatory drugs (Meloxicam, Piroxicam, Caprofen, ibuprofen, naproxen)	**Acute toxicity:** Anorexia, melena, frequent vomition, diarhhoea, abdominal pain **Chronic toxicity:** Weakness, hypotension, stumbling, pale mucous membranes, GI irritation, ulceration, perforations and hemorrhage, regenerative anemia, renal damage, CNS depression, ataxia, and seizures, increased BUN and creatinine, decreased total protein and increased bleeding time	• Alkalinization of the urine with sodium bicarbonate • Use of a proton-pump inhibitor • Use of sucralfate	Dog, cat

(4) Cough medications toxicity			
I) Antihistamines			
Chlorpheniramine, Dimenhydrinate, Diphenhydramine, Cetirizine	Hyperactivity or depression, hypersalivation, tachypnea, and tachycardia, vomition	• Induction of emesis in asymptomatic patients • Use of activated charcoal for recent ingestion • Use of Propranolol (0.02-0.06 mg/kg, IV) to treat consistent tachycardia in normotensive patients • Use of Diazepam to control seizures or seizure-type activity. Use of Physostigmine to counteract the CNS anticholinergic effects of antihistamine	Dog, cat
Clemestine	Sedation, lethargy, and anticholinergic signs (dry mouth, tachycardia, agitation, decreased intestinal secretions/motility)		
II) Dextromethorphan	CNS and GI effects such as agitation, hallucination, nervousness, mydriasis, shaking, vomiting, or diarrhea	• Use of Diazepam to control some of the CNS effects • Use of Phenothiazine tranquilizers (acepromazine or chlorpromazine) or cyproheptadine (1.1 mg/kg, PO or per rectum, for dogs, and 2–4 mg per cat; repeation in 6–8 hr if needed) for serotonin syndrome.	Dog, cat

5) Gastrointestinal drugs toxicity			
I) H_2-Receptor Antagonists **Cimetidine, famotidine, nizatidine, and ranitidine**	**Acute Oral overdoses:** vomiting, diarrhea, anorexia, and dry mouth. **Acute IV overdoses:** Tremors, hypotension, and bradycardia	• Symptomatic treatment • Fluid therapy	Dog, cat
II) Antacids (Calcium carbonate, aluminum hydroxide, and magnesium hydroxide (milk of magnesia))	Calcium- and aluminum-containing antacids generally cause constipation, whereas magnesium-containing antacids tend to cause diarrhea	• Induction of emesis within 2–3 hr of exposure may help prevent severe GI upset.	Dog, cat
(6) Vitamin toxicity			
I)Vitamin A	General malaise, anorexia, nausea, peeling skin, weakness, tremors, convulsions, paralysis		Dog
II) Vitamin D	Vomiting, depression, polyuria and polydipsia, and hyperphosphatemia may be seen within 12 hr of a significant vitamin D exposure, followed by hypercalcemia and acute renal failure		Dog
III) Vit K3	Renal colic, hematuria and renal failure in chronic cases		Horse
(7) Topical preparations toxicity (Zinc Oxide)	Facial and ocular edema		Dog

References

Garg, S. K. (2012). Veterinary toxicology. CBS Publishers & Distributors.
https://www.msdvetmanual.com/toxicology/toxicities-from-human-drugs.
Sandhu, H. S., and Brar, R. S. (2009). Textbook of veterinary toxicology. Kalyani publishers.

32

Chocolate Poisoning

Neelam Kushwaha

Key Points

- Dogs can be fed a wide variety of chocolate and cocoa-based goods, particularly during holiday seasons, such as candy, cakes, cookies, brownies, and chocolate chips.
- Dogs that eat chocolate usually become very sick, but they also seldom die from it.

Introduction

Caffeine and theobromine are found in chocolate. Dogs' metabolisms of caffeine and theobromine differ from humans'. Because they contain more theobromine and caffeine, darker, bitter chocolates are considered to be more dangerous.

When a dog consumes too much chocolate goods, it can lead to major health problems like seizures, heart failure, and muscular tremors. In extreme situations, the dog may even pass away from cardiac or respiratory failure. Due to the fat and sugar content, it induces vomiting and diarrhoea even in non-toxic doses. Numerous substances found in chocolate are hazardous to animals. Although chocolate poisoning can affect a wide variety of animal species, including dogs, cats, horses, and rodents, it most frequently affects dogs. Theobromine and caffeine are the main harmful ingredients in chocolate. The amount of caffeine and theobromine in chocolate varies with kind. Dogs' metabolism of theobromine and caffeine differs from that of humans. Dogs are more sensitive because of this. Dogs who consume chocolate may become seriously unwell, even though it rarely results in death. When a dog eats too many chocolate-containing foods, such as cakes, cookies, brownies, candies, and chocolate chips, it might become poisoned.

Dogs are more at risk from darker, more bitter chocolate. Chocolate contains fat and sugar, which can make dogs sick even at little doses that are not dangerous. These can result in pancreatitis in severe cases or in dogs with more sensitive stomachs.

Clinical signs

The following clinical indications are caused by chocolate's theobromine and caffeine content:

Signs related to the digestive system: Chocolate contains a lot of fat and sugar, which can lead to nausea and vomiting in any amount.

Consequences related to the heart, including arrhythmias, hypertension, and hypotension

Signs of the central nervous system include tremors, convulsions, agitation, pacing, and hyperactivity.

The type and quantity of chocolate the patient consumes determines the clinical symptoms. After consumption, clinical symptoms of chocolate toxicosis often manifest 2-4 hours later, though they may take up to 6-12 hours. The most typical clinical symptoms include diarrhea, vomiting, increased thirst, panting or restlessness, excessive urine, and tachycardia. Seizures, heart failure, and trembling of muscles occur in severe cases. Premature ventricular contractions, tachypnea, cyanosis, bradycardia, hypotension, hypertension, and coma are possible side effects. Heart failure may result from hypokalemia that develops later in the toxicosis. Respiratory failure, hyperthermia, and cardiac arrhythmias are the most frequent causes of mortality.

The prognosis for chocolate poisoning can deteriorate if complications such aspiratory pneumonia develop from aspiration during vomiting. Since clinical symptoms of chocolate poisoning might take many hours to manifest, prompt medical attention is recommended if a dangerously high quantity of chocolate is ingested. Long half-lives of theobromine allow for prolonged circulation retention; days may pass between symptoms following significant exposures.

Diagnosis

Diagnosis is made by history of ingestion of chocolate products. Clinical signs further aid in diagnosis.

Treatment

Stabilizing patients who are experiencing symptoms is the top goal when treating chocolate poisoning.

- Methocarbamol (50–220 mg/kg body weight, slow IV) or diazepam (0.5–2 mg/kg body weight, slow IV) may be administered for tremors and/or moderate seizures.
- The use of barbiturates or other general anesthetics may be necessary in cases with severe seizures.

Arrhythmias should only be addressed when absolutely required.

- Propranolol (0.02-0.06 mg/kg body weight, slow IV) or metoprolol (@ 0.2-0.4 mg/kg body weight, slow IV) are used to treat tachyarrhythmias.
- Bradyarrhythmia is treated with atropine (0.01-0.02 mg/kg body weight IV).

It is also possible for the bladder to reabsorb theobromine. In order to expedite the excretion of methylxanthines through the urine and regulate cardiovascular function, supportive therapies such as intravenous fluid therapy are recommended.

Only once a patient is stabilized or when clinical indications have not yet manifested (within an hour of consumption) may decontamination be carried out. To produce emesis, apomorphine or hydrogen peroxide administration should be initiated. Decontamination, which involves emesis inducement and the administration of activated charcoal to stop theobromine from being absorbed, is necessary if the patient receives treatment early. For as long as symptoms persist, patients should receive repeated doses of activated charcoal (1-4 g/kg, PO) due to the enterohepatic recirculation of methylxanthines (vomiting can be controlled with metoclopramide at 0.2-0.4 mg/kg, SC or IM, every 6 hours if required). Patients who have been put under sedation because of seizure activity may benefit from gastric lavage. An ECG should be performed to check the heart condition.

Correction of acid-base and electrolyte abnormalities, control of body temperature, and implantation of urinary catheters (methylxanthines and their metabolites can be reabsorbed through the bladder) are further treatments for patients exhibiting symptoms.

Key point for management of chocolate poisoning

1. Use activated charcoal to induce emesis or perform stomach lavage.
2. Observe the patient's vital indicators.
3. Intravenous hydration
4. If beta-blockers for tachycardia (such as propranolol and metoprolol)
5. Atropine if bradycardia
6. If anxiety appears, take diazepam
7. To maintain the bladder empty, catheterize the bladder and remove the urine catheter.

References

Knight, A. (2017). Chocolate Toxicity in Dogs, Cats, and Other Animals. Veterinary Clinics of North America: Small Animal Practice, 47(6), 1107-1126.

MSD Veterinary Manual. Chocolate Toxicosis in Animals. Available at: https://www.msdvetmanual.com/toxicology/food-hazards/chocolate-toxicosis-in-animals

Peetiya, N. (2023). Comprehensive Review of the Toxicity of Chocolate for Animals. International Journal of Healthcare Sciences, 11 (1): 26-27.

33

Metal and Non-Metal Toxicity

S. Ramanarayanan

Key Points

- It is frequently reported that metal, non-metal, and metalloid components cause toxicity in farm animals.
- The type of element causing toxicity affects both the treatment and the clinical indications of toxicity.
- The best course of action for managing toxicity is to treat symptoms first, then, if the causal toxin is known, use targeted antidotes.

Introduction

Animal diets contain a variety of environmental components, including metals and non-metals. Certain substances are necessary for the animal and only become poisonous when consumed in excess, while others simply endanger the animal's health. However, a number of variables, including the absorbed dose, the exposure route, the period of exposure (acute versus chronic), and others, affect how toxic the substance is, and these variables must be taken into account when diagnosing, treating, and managing clinical cases. Given the multitude of factors affecting these metals' toxicity. An attempt is made in this chapter to present a streamlined synopsis of the toxicity of metals, non-metals, and metalloid elements that are frequently encountered.

Lead Toxicity

Source

Lead is infamous for being one of the components that veterinary doctors face poisoning from the most frequently [1]. The main source of toxicity, especially in young children, is lead that is released into the environment through incorrect disposal of old batteries, smelting of lead ores, welding, soldering, and other activities; unintentional ingestion of motor oils, grease, or other farm automobile products; and lead excreted through the milk of lead-poisoned animals.

Toxicity

It has been observed that acute oral exposure to lead at a body weight of 200–400 mg/kg in calves and 600–800 mg/kg in cattle can be fatal [2]. On the other hand, horses were shown to be toxic when exposed to lead at a daily dose of 1.7 mg/kg body weight (1). The FDA established a maximum allowable limit of 10 ppm for lead [3].

Clinical signs

Nervous system and gastrointestinal problems are among the most common clinical indicators of poisoning. Within 24 to 48 hours, ataxia, muscle spasms, teeth bruxing, blindness, muscle tremors, convulsions, and eventually death are the symptoms of acute poisoning. The symptoms of acute poisoning in horses include roaring and laryngeal paralysis. Chronic lead poisoning in animals typically manifests as nonspecific clinical symptoms such diarrhea, stomach pain, gastrointestinal disorders (including cessation of rumination), anorexia, lethargy, weight loss, and behavioral abnormalities like hyperesthesia [1,4].

Diagnosis

Prominent post-mortem abnormalities include cerebral cortex congestion with flattening of the cortical gyri, oedema, renal tubular necrosis, and gastroenteritis [5]. Lead concentrations of 0.35 ppm in blood and 10 ppm in organs like the kidney and liver are frequently used as diagnostic indicators for lead poisoning.

Treatment

The toxic effects can be mitigated by treatment with certain chelating agents, such as calcium disodium ethylenediaminetetraacetic acid (Ca-EDTA), administered via slow IV or SC twice daily for three days at a dose of 110 mg/kg body weight in calves (1-2% solution in 5% DNS) and 25 mg/kg body weight in dogs [2,5]. If necessary, the treatment may be given again two days later. Ca-EDTA can be nephrotoxic, hence caution should be used when giving it to animals, especially those that are dehydrated. Dimercaprol and Ca-EDTA together can also be utilized, but use caution. Thiamine (Vitamin B1) injections at a dose of 2 mg/kg intramuscularly or subcutaneously (SC) and magnesium sulfate baths are examples of supportive care [6]. N-acetylcysteine (50 mg/kg/day, PO), an antioxidant, has also been found to have positive effects [5]. When required, symptomatic therapy is recommended. Animal bones and milk with lead residues pose a risk to public health.

Mercury Toxicity

Source

Mercury is another metal that comes in several chemical forms: elemental (like light bulbs and thermometers), inorganic (like latex paints and batteries) and organic (like aryl, methyl, or ethyl) mercury salts. There are a number of potential sources of mercury toxicity, including contaminated feed (fish meal, for example), natural sources (such as groundwater, metal ores, and metal leaching from the soil) [7].

Toxicity and clinical signs

The form of mercury exposed, the route of exposure, and a number of other factors affect the toxicokinetics of mercury, although generally speaking, organo-mercurial compounds are thought to be more dangerous. Organo-mercurial poisoning primarily manifests as neurological symptoms such as ataxia, visual abnormalities, tremors in the muscles, and paralysis, which are followed by coma and death. On the other hand, the inorganic salts of mercury are very caustic and seriously harm the mucosal lining of the stomach, resulting in stomatitis, enteritis, regurgitation, and hemorrhagic diarrhea, which in turn causes electrolyte and fluid loss, hypovolemic shock, and fatality [2,7,8].

Diagnosis

Mercury concentrations in blood, tissue, and feed issue samples of less than 1 ppm or 0.1 mg/kg are regarded as normal [2,9]. In contrast, acute poisoning cases can show blood levels of >6 mg/kg, 10 mg/kg in the kidneys, and 0.5 mg/kg in the brain [9]. The main methods of diagnosis are clinical manifestations and a patient's history of exposure; mercury levels in the blood and kidneys are then checked.

Treatment

General, targeted, and supportive therapy are all part of the treatment plan. Oral administration of sodium thiosulfate (0.5–1 g/kg) and activated charcoal (1-3 g/kg) will bind mercury and prevent absorption. It is advised to chelate the heavy metal in large animals by injecting 3 mg/kg of dimercaprol (British Anti-lewisite; BAL) deep intraperitoneally every 4 hours for the first two days, every 6 hours on the third day, and twice daily for the following ten days [2,10]. BAL should not be administered to those who have a history of renal or hepatic illness. For chelation, oral agents such mesodimercaptosuccinic acid (DMSA) (10 mg/kg) or D-penicillamine (15–50 mg/kg) might be used.

Chelation agents require careful dosage management because an incorrect dose can cause therapy to fail and an overdose can be harmful. To improve elimination, companion animals may benefit from the use of plasma exchange-hemodialysis-plasma pheresis [7]. Since organic mercury can build up in the body and pose a risk to public health and food safety, euthanasia and proper disposal of animal carcasses should be carried out.

Arsenic Toxicity

Source

The three major types of arsenic found in nature are elemental (As3), trivalent (As3+), and pentavalent (As5+). While many of the poisonous sources have been replaced throughout time, arsenic poisoning is still primarily caused by volcanic eruptions, contaminated ground water, smelting of ores, etc. These sources are still present in emerging nations. Exposure can occur through ingestion, inhalation, or skin contact and can be acute, sub-acute, or chronic.

Toxicity and clinical signs

For most species, a dose of sodium arsenite of one to 25 mg/kg is thought to be fatal. While a total dose of arsenic trioxide is thought to be fatal at 10-45 g for horses, 15-45 g for cattle, and 3-10 g for sheep and goats. In situations of acute toxicity of trivalent mercurials, the symptoms include severe colic, vomiting, gastroenteritis, diarrhea, unsteady gait, collapse, paralysis, and animal death. Pentavalent arsenical toxicity manifests neurologically as incoordination, weakening of the muscles, and a seated dog posture; in animals, it manifests as blindness, paralysis, and recumbency.

Diagnosis and treatment

The diagnosis of arsenic toxicity is provisional and dependent on clinical indications, lesions, history of exposure, and circumstantial evidence; confirmation of the diagnosis is obtained by the identification of arsenic in ingested materials and tissues. IV fluids are the first line of treatment, and then symptomatic treatments. It is recommended to use activated charcoal to absorb the arsenic in dogs and cats and to induce emesis in conscious animals [11]. Chelating agents: utilize D-penicillamine, DMSA, or dimercaprol (BAL) sparingly, as dosage needs to be carefully considered.

Copper Toxicity

Source

The diagnosis of arsenic toxicity is provisional and dependent on clinical indications, lesions, history of exposure, and circumstantial evidence; confirmation of the diagnosis is obtained by the identification of arsenic in ingested materials and tissues. IV fluids are the first line of treatment, and then symptomatic treatments. It is recommended to use activated charcoal to absorb the arsenic in dogs and cats and to induce emesis in conscious animals [11]. Chelating agents: utilize D-penicillamine, DMSA, or dimercaprol (BAL) sparingly, as dosage needs to be carefully considered.

Toxicity and clinical signs

Sheep are often more vulnerable to copper toxicity due to their propensity to collect copper in the liver more quickly than other animal species [1,2]. The severity of copper toxicity varies depending on the animal species, breed, kind of chemical exposed to, etc. Toxic amounts of copper are defined as exceeding 250 ppm, 40 ppm in cattle, and 25 ppm in sheep (2). Abdominal pain, hypersalivation, gastroenteritis, greenish-tinged diarrhea, hematemesis, shock, and death are examples of clinical indications of poisoning. After an early period of gastrointestinal upset, animals that survive exhibit hemolysis and hemoglobinuria.

Diagnosis and treatment

Kidneys that are bluish black in color and sometimes referred to as "gun metal kidneys" are unusual post-mortem discoveries made in animals who have died from copper intoxication. Copper toxicity also manifests as icteric liver, enlarged gall bladder, erosions, ulcers in the ruminant abomasum, and splenomegaly. Confirmatory evidence is provided by blueish-green-tinged ingesta and elevated serum and tissue (kidney, liver) copper levels [1]. To improve the removal of copper, oral chelating drugs such D-Penicillamine (10–15 mg/kg) might be employed. In cases of severe copper toxicity, blood transfusions may be recommended. Antioxidant therapy with Vitamin E (400–500 mg/kg) [2], oral zinc supplementation (5–10 mg/kg), and molybdenum fortification of diets may all aid in supportive therapy. Copper absorption may also be prevented.

Molybdenum Toxicity

Source

Molybdenum is another significant trace mineral that functions as a co-factor for a number of biological enzymes. A feed mismatch between copper and molybdenum frequently causes the toxicity.

Toxicity and clinical signs

Ingestion of plants cultivated on polluted soils or soil types that are typically rich in molybdenum or contaminated with mining or smeltery waste are the main causes of toxicity. A copper:molybdenum ratio of less than 2:1 in feed is suggestive of poisoning. The animals that are afflicted display symptoms such as anorexia, restlessness, and severe watery diarrhea with gas bubbles called "peat scours or teart," which can cause acute episodes of generalized weakness, shock, and even death. On the other hand, signs of sub-acute and chronic molybdenum toxicity may be similar to those of copper deficiency, where a weakening of the heart is caused by gradual myocardial atrophy. After physical effort or exercise, the animal may collapse and die; this illness is known as falling disease in cattle.

Buffaloes can have focal or generalized skin depigmentation, whereas sheep can have enzootic ataxia, also known as sway back, which is the paralysis of the hind quarters brought on by demyelination of nerves. Microcytic hypochromic anemia arises from a haematological perspective. The non-specific postmortem abnormalities include bleeding, diarrhea, and degenerative alterations to the kidney and liver. Changes in the relative concentrations of copper and molybdenum in feed and tissues (liver and kidney) can provide confirmation.

Treatment consists of removing molybdenum-containing foods from the diet, adding copper to the diet, and adjusting the copper-to-molybdenum ratio. It is possible to administer injectable copper compounds [12], such as copper glycinate at 120 mg/cow SC (12). It has also been demonstrated that lowering the symptoms can be achieved by adding copper sulphate at a rate of 1-2 g/ adult cow or by using copper sulphate salt licks [2].

Fluoride Toxicity

Source

Fluoride is a common non-metal element that is extensively dispersed and highly reactive. One of the most pervasive issues in India and many other developing nations is fluorine poisoning. In many cases, the main cause of fluorosis is drinking water tainted with high fluorine levels [13]. In addition to drinking water, other sources of fluorosis include the usage of mineral fertilizers high in fluoride, industrial effluents, etc.

Toxicity and clinical signs

Since fluoride toxicity develops gradually over time, it can be mistaken for other chronic illnesses such degenerative arthritis. Lameness, an excruciatingly painful stride, and skeletal abnormalities, including ribcage, sternum, and mandible enlargement, are evident; scoliosis, joint and limb swelling, spontaneous bone fractures, cachexia, and death ensue. Teeth exhibiting distinctive mottling and patchy dentine loss are signs of dental fluorosis [1]. In extreme situations, dental tables might distort and teeth can fall out.

Diagnosis and treatment

The diagnosis of fluorosis is based on clinical indicators, measurement of fluoride levels in feed and water, and X-ray examination of sick animals. It is possible to test the fluoride concentration of tooth ash or bone ash; in addition to bone and teeth, urine and plasma can also have high fluoride levels. When it comes to acute poisoning, the prognosis is dire; in chronic cases, hypocalcaemia can be treated with intravenous calcium administration, dialysis to eliminate excess fluorine, removing the animal from toxicity sources, and supportive therapy involving fluids, analgesics, and antibiotics to relieve symptoms [1, 2, 13].

Selenium Toxicity

Source

In trace quantities (0.1–0.3 ppm), selenium is a necessary non-metal for maintaining normal health. On the other hand, an excess of either organic or inorganic selenium—from plants that store selenium, tainted drinking water, industrial effluent, etc.—causes toxicosis. Selenium poisoning in animals is also frequently caused by an accidental overdose that occurs during the delivery of injectable or oral supplements [14].

Toxicity and clinical signs

Selenium has a 0.1–0.3 ppm dietary requirement, while 1–5 ppm is the maximum dosage that livestock, sheep, and horses can tolerate. Selenium levels above 5 parts per million in feed pose a serious risk to ruminants [2]. Oral dosages of 1–5 mg/kg Se cause acute toxicity. Lethargy, colic, bloat, dyspnea, watery diarrhea, weak and rapid heartbeats, unconsciousness, and death within 1-2 days are the symptoms of acute selenium intoxication. The symptoms of sub-acute selenium toxicity/blind staggers include the animal walking into objects, leg weakness, paralysis of the tongue and throat, and eventually death.

Animals with chronic selenium toxicity (also known as alkali disease) exhibit lameness, stiff gait, hoof cracking and sloughing, hair coat loss, apathy, and emaciation. Severe circumstances may also show gangrenous alterations in the limbs, which might result in septicemia.

Diagnosis and treatment

Selenium levels in blood can reach up to 25 ppm in acute cases and up to 4 ppm in chronic situations. Selenium levels in tissue, such as the kidney and liver, range from 4 to 25 ppm, in urine from 0.1 to 8 ppm, and in milk from 1-3 ppm (2). The animal's hoof, hair, and wool may also contain selenium in cases of chronic selenosis and can be useful for diagnosis. Although there isn't a known cure for selenium poisoning, there are several recommended treatments to manage the symptoms, such as fluid therapy to prevent diarrhoea and hypovolemic shock, purgatives to eliminate unabsorbed selenium, and acetyl cysteine to replace depleted glutathione.

Sodium Chloride (Salt) Poisoning

Source

Common salt, also known as sodium chloride, is a necessary part of an animal's diet because it helps the body perform biological processes including nerve impulse transmission and osmotic equilibrium maintenance by supplying sodium and chloride ions. Animal diets often include 0.5–1% sodium chloride in addition to extra access to salt blocks. Animals that have access to fresh water can withstand high salt concentrations. However, salt sickness can result from consuming too much salt or from being dehydrated.

Toxicity and clinical signs

While dogs and cats can withstand salt levels of 3.7% in their diet when they have access to fresh water, swine are said to be more susceptible to salt toxicity, with an acute hazardous dosage of about 2.2 g/kg [15, 16]. Clinical signs include increased thirst, loss of appetite, gastroenteritis, increased osmolarity in cerebrospinal fluid (which causes cerebral oedema), and symptoms such as aimless wandering, circling, head pressing, etc. Cattle have also been reported to experience blindness, seizures, and paralysis [15]. Brain oedema, ulceration and bleeding in the gastrointestinal tract, and gastroenteritis are examples of post-mortem lesions.

Diagnosis and treatment

Increased sodium concentrations in the blood and over 2000 parts per million in the brain are thought to be diagnostically significant. As part of the treatment, patients are encouraged to drink 0.5% of their body weight in water every hour until they are fully rehydrated. Fluid therapy in the form of 5% dextrose solution and furosemide at 3.7 mL/kg/h as a diuretic should be administered [15]. Mannitol is recommended as a therapy for cerebral edema.

References

1. Thompson LJ. Metals and Micronutrients. In: Gupta RC, editor. Veterinary Toxicology, Basic and Clinical Principles. 3rd ed. United States: Academic Press, Elsevier Inc.; 2018. p. 439–42.
2. Sandhu HS, Brar RS. Textbook of Veterinary Toxicology. 2nd ed. Sandhu HS, Brar RS, editors. New Delhi: Kalyani Publishers; 2009. 101–177 p.
3. FDA-CVM. CVM CY15-17 Report on Heavy Metals in Animal Food [Internet]. 2011. Available from: https://www.fda.gov/media/132046/download
4. Cowan V, Blakley B. Acute lead poisoning in western Canadian cattle - A 16-year retrospective study of diagnostic case records. Can Vet J. 2016;57(4):421–6.

5. Blakley BR. Lead Poisoning in Animals. MSD Veterinary Manual. 2022. Available from: https://www.msdvetmanual.com/toxicology/lead-poisoning/lead-poisoning-in-animals
6. California Department of Food & Agriculture. Lead Toxicity and its Effects on Animals and Animal Products. 2016;(July):9350. Available from: https://www.cdfa.ca.gov/ahfss/Animal_Health/pdfs/leadtoxicity.pdf
7. Neustadt J, Pieczenik S. Heavy-metal toxicity - With emphasis on mercury. Integr Med. 2007;6(2):26–32.
8. Liu J, Goyer RA, Waalkes MP. Toxic Effects of Metals. In: Klaassen CD, editor. Casarett and Doull's Toxicology The Basic Science of Poisons. 7th ed. New york; 2008. p. 931–80.
9. Blakley BR. Mercury Poisoning in Animals. MSD Veterinary Manual. 2022. Available from:https://www.msdvetmanual.com/toxicology/mercury-poisoning/mercury-poisoning-in-animals
10. Gupta RC, Milatovic D, Lall R, Srivastava A. Mercury. In: Gupta RC, editor. Veterinary Toxicology, Basic and Clinical Principles. 3rd ed. United States: Academic Press, Elsevier Inc.; 2018. p. 455–60.
11. Garland T. Inorganic Arsenical Toxicosis in Animals. MSD Veterinary Manual. 2022. Availablefrom:https://www.msdvetmanual.com/toxicology/arsenicpoisoning/inorganic-arsenical-toxicosis-in-animals
12. Blakley BR. Molybdenum Toxicity in Animals. MSD Veterinary Manual. 2022. Available from: https://www.msdvetmanual.com/toxicology/molybdenum-toxicity/molybdenum-toxicity-in-animals
13. Choubisa SL. Status of Fluorosis in Animals. Proc Natl Acad Sci India Sect B Biol Sci. 2012;82(3):331–9. Available from: https://doi.org/10.1007/s40011-012-0026-0
14. Hall JO. Selenium. In: Gupta RC, editor. Veterinary Toxicology, Basic and Clinical Principles. 3rd ed. United States: Academic Press, Elsevier Inc.; 2018. p. 470–7.
15. Thompson LJ. Sodium Chloride (Salt). In: Gupta RC, editor. Veterinary Toxicology, Basic and Clinical Principles. 3rd ed. United States: Academic Press, Elsevier Inc.; 2018. p. 479–82.
16. NRC. Mineral Tolerance of Animals. Second Rev. Washington D.C.: National Research Counsil, National Academies Press; 2005. 357–371 p.

34

Pesticide Poisoning

Safeeda Sultana Begum

Key Points

- When pesticides, which are chemicals used to manage a pest, impact non-target organisms like humans and animals, it's known as pesticide poisoning.
- Pesticides have the ability to contaminate the surrounding area and the ecosystem.

Introduction

Pesticides are chemical chemicals that are applied to destroy pests. These insecticides have the capacity to contaminate the surrounding area and the ecosystem. Pesticides can also be hazardous to a wide range of other creatures, including fish, birds, beneficial insects, and non-target plants, in addition to having a toxic effect on insects and weeds.

Etiology

Today's society faces several issues due to the overuse of pesticides in fields and food. Products may deteriorate if they are kept in partially filled containers for extended periods of time or exposed, whether intentionally or unintentionally, to high temperatures. It is dangerous to store chemicals anywhere other than their original container since the identification and label instructions are lost. These products can have severe effects on people or animals if they come into unintended touch with them. It can be extremely risky to mix substances or use them in unapproved combinations. In order to increase the efficacy of certain pesticide formulations, such as pyrethrins, pyrethroids, and d-limonene, piperonyl butoxide is added. It lessens the chemical's breakdown in the body of the insect or animal, but it also increases the pesticide's toxicity to both the pest and the host animal.

Clinical indicators

After exposure, poisoning symptoms could appear a few hours later. Excessive drooling, slight tremors, incoordination, excitability, or depression are examples of nervous system symptoms. More seriously impacted animals may experience convulsions, severe tremors, and respiratory failure leading to death.

Conclusion

Based on clinical manifestations, exposure history, and the discovery of pesticide residues in bodily fluids and tissues via a biopsy or postmortem, it is determined.

Treatment

The initial line of action should be to extract the toxin from the animal. If the animal consumed the product or a similar contaminated product less than two hours prior, vomiting should be instigated right away. If the animal is depressed, it is not advisable to induce vomiting; instead, a particular treatment should be administered in accordance with the pesticide's antidote requirements. For instance, atropine and pralidoxime, often known as 2 PAM, the antidote, are used to reverse organophosphate poisoning symptoms. Should the animal have skin exposure from pesticides, a mild detergent and water wash should be administered. When taken orally, mineral oil reduces the amount of the substance that is absorbed from the digestive system. Another useful substance is activated charcoal, which is regarded as a universal antidote. It might be necessary to administer oxygen or perform artificial respiration. Giving tranquilizers is not a good idea.

Precaution

It's crucial to always follow the label's instructions on how to use pesticides since they provide information on how to do so. Warnings against using on unapproved species or in testing conditions must also be included on labels. A maximum of care should be made to prevent drift or drainage to neighbouring fields, pastures, ponds, streams, or other properties outside the treatment area. In no case should amounts larger than those specifically recommended be utilized.

References

https://www.msdvetmanual.com/respiratory-system/non-infectious-respiratory-system-diseases-in-cattle/hypersensitivity-pneumonitis-in-cattle.

Micheal Taiwo Ayankoso, Damilola miracle Oluwagbamila, Olugbenga Samson ABE (2023). Effects of activated charcoal on livestock production: A review. Slovak Journal of Animal Science, 56 (1): 46–60

Radostits, O. M., Gay, C. C., Blood, D. C. & Hinchcliff, K. W. (2000). Veterinary Medicine: A textbook of cattle, sheep, pigs, goats and horses, nona edizione. Saunders, London, UK.

35

Plant Toxicity

S. Ramanarayanan

Key Points

- It might be necessary to administer oxygen or perform artificial respiration. Giving tranquilizers is not a good idea.
- Precaution: It's crucial to always follow the label's instructions on how to use pesticides since they provide information on how to do so. Warnings against using on unapproved species or in testing conditions must also be included on labels. A maximum of care should be made to prevent drift or drainage to neighboring fields, pastures, ponds, streams, or other properties outside the treatment area. In no case should amounts larger than those specifically recommended be utilized.

Introduction

It has been determined that a number of plant species are poisonous to animals. These plants not only posed a health risk to humans and animals, but they also significantly reduced cattle productivity. Many plants contain chemicals that can be dangerous or even lethal to animals. The degree of toxicity varies based on the animal species, the quantity of plant material ingested, and the particular poisonous compounds in question. In general, there are two categories of dangerous plants: those that are known to be toxic and contain toxic compounds, and those that are normally non-toxic but can turn hazardous in certain circumstances. Here are some typical plant toxicities, along with information on managing toxicity and clinical signs.

Plants Causing Cyanide Poisoning

Source

Plants classified as cyanogenic include cyanogenic glycosides, which when consumed by animals cause the production of hydrogen cyanide (HCN). Sorghum (jowar), Sudan grass, sugarcane (tops and leaves), eucalyptus, Lin seed, velvet grass, wild clove, bitter almond, and wild cherry are among the commonly found plants that are toxic [1,2].

Toxicity and clinical signs

Because ruminal microbiota helps convert cyanogenic glycosides into HCN, ruminants are more vulnerable. The amount of cyanogenic glycosides is dependent on a number of variables, including the plant's age and portion, the weather, when the plant is cut, the composition of the soil, the usage of fertilizers, etc. Toxicological symptoms are severe, and death usually happens in two hours. Anxiety, restlessness, bright red mucous membranes, dyspnea, a weak and fast pulse, convulsions, and respiratory paralysis are among the symptoms displayed by affected animals [3].

Diagnosis and treatment

A sodium picrate paper test can be used to examine the suspected contents of the ruminant at the field level in addition to the history, clinical indicators, and unusual bitter almond odor breath in making the diagnosis. Samples that should be transported to the lab in airtight containers under refrigerated circumstances include liver, muscles, rumen or stomach contents, and heparinized whole blood. Cyanide poisoning has a specialized treatment that needs to start right away. The contents of one 0.3-mL vial of amyl nitrite can be forced into the animal's mouth as soon as it is exposed [2]. It involves slowly injecting 20 mg/kg of sodium nitrite and 500 mg/kg of sodium thiosulfate intravenously to cattle [1]. To stop the creation of HCN, the rumen can be acidified and cooled using a 20% acetic acid solution in cold water. Treatment that is supportive and symptomatic is suggested.

Plants Causing Nitrate Poisoning

Source

The creation of macromolecules like DNA, RNA, proteins, hormones, and enzymes is one of the many biological activities that depend on nitrogen. Plants supply most of the nitrogen found in all living systems, mostly in the form of nitrate (NO3-), which the body then converts to nitrite (NO2-) for use later. Nitrate poisoning is caused by feeding nitrate-rich forages (such as alfalfa, sunflower, rye, sorghum, maize, soybeans, wheat, etc.) or plants that have received high nitrogen fertilizer dosages. Rich sources of nitrates include sewage, decomposing organic stuff like plant or animal waste, and industrial effluents. Nitrate toxicity is seen when they affect pasture lands or sources of drinking water.

Toxicity and clinical signs

By contrast, the nitrate ion is less hazardous since it is less reactive than the nitrite ion. Cattle are thought to be fatally exposed to sodium nitrate at a dosage rate of approximately 650–850 mg/kg body weight, whereas the lethal dose of sodium nitrite is 150–170 mg/kg body weight [4].Increased salivation, abdominal pain, gastroenteritis, diarrhea, rapid breathing rate as a major symptom, generalized muscular weakness, ataxia, open mouth breathing, collapse, and death are all indications of nitrite poisoning that can manifest as early as 30 minutes after administration. Methaemoglobin production gives blood its characteristic chocolate brown color.

Diagnosis and treatment

Based on clinical indications and a history of contact with nitrate-rich plants, a provisional diagnosis can be formed. Estimating the nitrate/nitrite content in dietary samples, plasma, or the aqueous humour of the eye can be used to make a confirmation diagnosis. When sending the samples to the lab, they must be collected in airtight containers and kept refrigerated. Specific antidotes, such as methylene blue at 4–8 mg/kg body weight in sheep and cattle and 5–10 mg/kg slow IV in dogs, are used as part of the treatment [4]. The use of cold water for rumen lavage, purgatives to improve nitrite excretion, oxygen therapy, and blood transfusions are examples of supportive therapy and care.

Plants Causing Photosensitization

The development of aberrant sensitivity in the skin's weakly pigmented patches to ultraviolet radiation or sunshine is known as photosensitization. The presence of a photodynamic substance in the peripheral circulation causes this severe type of dermatitis. There are two types of this condition: primary and secondary photosensitization. Several plants, some of which are covered here, can cause this condition.

a. *Primary photosensitization*

Here, the photoreactive chemical enters the peripheral circulation directly from the plant, primarily in its original form. After then, it combines with UV rays or ambient light to produce photodermatitis. Fagopyrum esculentum (buckweed), which contains fagopyrin, and Hypericium perforatum (Saint John's wort or Klamath weed), which includes the photoreactive chemical hypericin, are two significant plants implicated in primary photosensitization. Ayurvedic medicines frequently use several plants, many of which are thought to have therapeutic properties [5]. In addition to plants, phenothiazine, sulphonamides, and tetracyclines are examples of chemical agents that can induce primary photosensitization.

b. *Secondary photosensitization*

This is the most prevalent type of photosensitization and is sometimes referred to as hepatogenous photosensitization [6]. In this case, the photodynamic agent is phylloerythrin, which is created, especially in ruminants, following the breakdown of chlorophyll. Normally formed, phylloerythrin enters the bloodstream, undergoes conjugation metabolism in the liver, and is eliminated by bile. However, the phylloerythrin penetrates peripheral circulation and causes photosensitization in cases of liver injury or biliary obstruction. widespread causes include the widespread decorative plant Lantana camara, also known as Raimuniya in Hindi or common lantana, because of its lovely blossoms.

Clinical signs

Similar clinical symptoms are seen in photosensitization regardless of kind. whereby animals that are light-sensitive become uncomfortable when exposed to light. Photosensitization is more common in areas where there is less hair cover. It starts as skin irritation and progresses to erythema, pruritis, and painful, oedematous swelling of the affected area. If light exposure is avoided at this point, the symptoms go away quickly; if light exposure is allowed to continue, necrosis, ulceration, serum exudation from the lesion, and sloughing of the skin follow, all of which can result in subsequent bacterial infection. Liver damage, anorexia, jaundice, weight loss, and ascites are seen if photosensitization is secondary [1].

Diagnosis and treatment

One distinctive indication that can aid in diagnosis is dermatitis restricted to the non-pigmented area. The categorization of jaundice types is aided by serum examination for indicators of liver damage and jaundice. Animals receiving treatment are taken off of feed that contains plants or photoactive materials. corticosteroid administration to reduce dermatitis. When treating secondary bacterial infections, use antibiotics. Secondary photosensitization can be aided by administering hepatoprotective medications (such as silymarin) after receiving fluid and electrolyte therapy.

Plants Causing Oxalate Poisoning

Oxalates, which are salts of sodium, ammonium, calcium, magnesium, and potassium, are accumulated by plants such Beta vulgaris (sugar beat), Halogeton glomeratus, and oxalis pescaprae. Because some plants are edible, eating them in big amounts can make them hazardous. Up to 650 g of oxalic acid can be tolerated by cattle and buffaloes [4], however sheep fed on pasture containing 2% sodium or potassium oxalates may die.

Following absorption, oxalate binds to either magnesium or calcium in the blood, resulting in hypomagnesemia or hypocalcaemia. In chronic poisoning situations, oxalate crystals build up in the renal tubules, blood vessels, and rumen epithelium, leading to renal necrosis. Acute poisoning episodes can include anorexia, weakness, hemorrhages from compromised clotting, incoordination, and paralysis. Hypocalcemia is the primary cause of the clinical symptoms. In addition to the history and clinical symptoms, the presence of oxalate crystals in the kidneys and oxalate in probable feed should help with the diagnosis. The recommended course of treatment entails giving suspected fodder no more food, administering lime water (Ca[OH]2), and occasionally, but not always, giving injectable calcium to address hypocalcemia.

Plants Causing Selenium Poisoning

When compared to other plants, some have a tendency to accumulate selenium from the soil; these plants are categorized as obligatory accumulators, facultative accumulators, and non-accumulator plants. As examples, consider:

i) Provide selenium accumulators: Because these plants need selenium to flourish, they are more likely to accumulate it. These plants can have selenium contents ranging from 100 to 15,000 ppm [1].

   For example: Astragalus species, Onopsis species, and Xylorrhiza species.

ii) Facultative selenium accumulators: Although these plants can accumulate selenium up to 25–100 ppm, they do not need it for growth.

   such as Astriplex species, Aster species, etc.

iii) Non-accumulator plants: When cultivated in soils high in selenium, these plants have the ability to collect selenium.

For instance: Barley, wheat, and maize.Animals who consume these plants when there is a drought typically become poisonous to selenium.

Datura Poisoning

Atropa belladonna (deadly nightshade), Hyoscyamus niger (black henbane), Datura stramonium (Jimson weed or devil's trumpet), and other plants have glycol-alkaloids, which are toxic compounds, such as atropine, hyoscine (scopolamine), or daturine.Although poisoning is rare because the plants are usually unattractive and inedible, toxicity can occasionally result from eating on these plants during a drought or by inadvertently ingesting the seeds. The symptoms of atropine overdose are similar to those of datura and related plant poisoning. Symptoms of poisoning may include mydriasis, cycloplegia, motor incoordination, dry mouth, hallucinations, and stumbling gait. The history, clinical indicators, and circumstantial evidence are used to make the diagnosis. taking activated charcoal orally to clean the stomach, then using the parasympathomimetic medication physostigmine to treat the clinical symptoms of toxicity is advised.

Oleander and Other Cardiotoxic Plants

This comprises plants that contain toxic glycosides that are poisonous to animals, such as digitoxin, oleandrin, and Asclepias spp. (milkweed), Nerium odorum (white oleander), and Digitalis purpurea (foxglove plant). Among these, Nerium odorum is a popular ornamental plant whose leaves can become poisonous if they come into contact with animal feed by accident.As a result of the poisonous glycosides' action on the heart, asystole and electrical conductivity are blocked by inhibiting the sodium potassium pump, or Na+/K+-ATPase [7]. While large doses result in arrhythmia, conduction abnormalities, reduced cardiac output, and mortality within 24 hours of the beginning of clinical symptoms, lower levels have a favorable ionotropic effect. It is recommended to do early gastrointestinal cleansing using purgatives, activated charcoal, and emesis induction.

Plants Causing Lathyrism

The disease known as lathyrism is brought on by eating legumes from the genus Lathyrus, which includes wild peas. Plants like Lathyrus odoratus (sweet pea), L. sativus (grass pea or khesari dal), L. Latifolius, and others are included in it. Osteolathyrism and neurolathyrism are the two primary categories of lathyrism. While neurolathyrism is less common [1] and is characterized by generalized muscular weakness, shifting lameness, stiff gait, respiratory muscle paralysis, and death, the toxic principle involved in osteolathyrism is primarily observed in cattle and is characterized by lameness of the hind limbs, exostoses, and pain in the feet. The primary diagnostic tools are circumstantial evidence and clinical indicators. It is recommended to combine supportive care with symptomatic therapy.

Plants Producing Thiamine Deficiency

An enzyme known as thiaminase is found in some plants, including Pteridium aquilinum (bracken fern or eagle fern), Equisetum arvense (horsetail or saapghas in Hindi), etc. This enzyme catalyzes the breakdown of thiamine (Vitamin B1), leading to a vitamin B1 shortage. When these plants are consumed in large quantities, the toxicity they generate is comparable to thiamine deficiency. In addition to thiaminase, these plants also contain poisonous principles such haematuria factor (which produces enzootic hemorrhages) and ptaquiloside (which suppresses bone marrow and causes aplastic anemia).

Clinical manifestations include neurological symptoms such hemoglobinuria, muscle tremors, stumbling gait, incoordination, clonic spasms, and death. It was reported that blood pyruvate levels were rising while blood thiamine levels were falling [1]. Animals should not be allowed to feed on polluted pastures in cases of early diagnosis. Instead, treatment with thiamine injection at a dose of 5 mg/kg body weight via IV or IM route has reported to be effective.

References

1. Sandhu HS, Brar RS. Poisonous Plants. In: Sandhu HS, Brar RS, editors. Textbook of Veterinary Toxicology. 2nd ed. New Delhi: Kalyani Publishers; 2009. p. 283–313.
2. Cope RB. Cyanide Poisoning in Animals. MSD Veterinary Manual. 2022. Available from:https://www.msdvetmanual.com/toxicology/cyanide-poisoning/cyanide-poisoning-in-animals
3. Stoltenow C, Lardy G. Understanding Cyanide Poisoning. North Dakota State University Extension. 2020;1150(May). Available from: https://www.ag.ndsu.edu/publications/livestock/cyanide-poisoning
4. Sandhu HS, Brar RS. Textbook of Veterinary Toxicology. 2nd ed. Sandhu HS, Brar RS, editors. New Delhi: Kalyani Publishers; 2009. 101–177 p.
5. Sonani S, Dudhamal TS. Pharmacological activity of Ayurveda herbal medicines in anxiety and depression : A review. J Drug Res Ayurvedic Sci. 2023;8:113–23.
6. Panter KE, Welch KD, Gardner DR, Lee ST, Green BT, Pfister JA, et al. Poisonous Plants of the United States. In: Gupta RC, editor. Veterinary Toxicology, Basic and Clinical Principles. 3rd ed. United States: Academic Press, Elsevier Inc.; 2018. p. 837–89.
7. Gupta PK. Chapter 21 - Toxic effects of cardiac poisons. In: Gupta PK, editor. Fundamentals of Toxicology. Academic Press; 2016. p. 245–51. Available from: https://www.sciencedirect.com/science/article/pii/B9780128054260000214

36

Urea Poisoning

S. Ramanarayanan

Key Points

- With the aid of microorganisms, ruminants typically use NPN to synthesis proteins for nutritional needs.
- When there is an excess of urea in the body, ammonia is produced excessively, which can be harmful.
- The majority of clinical indicators are neurological in nature, and their severity varies depending on a number of variables.
- Ruminal environment acidification to stop excessive ammonia generation and absorption; symptomatic therapy is advised.

Introduction

In addition to being a widely utilized fertilizer for crops, urea is frequently used in animal feeds as a low-cost protein substitute [1]. The previously mentioned explanations explain the reports of urea toxicity in ruminants. These animals may use non-protein nitrogen (NPN) like urea to create ammonia, which is subsequently used to synthesize proteins that partially meet their nutritional needs. This is made possible by the urease enzyme and ruminal microorganisms. On the other hand, rapid overconsumption of NPN leads to excessive ammonia generation and toxicity. This chapter aims to provide an overview of some of the most frequent causes of urea poisoning, clinical symptoms to watch out for, and associated treatments.

Toxicity

Animals that are starving are more susceptible to urea toxicity than those that are fed well, and the most common causes of urea poisoning are sudden diet changes to urea or exposure to urea-treated feed [3]. Adult sheep and cattle that are fed high-urea diets without having previously adapted are often more vulnerable to the toxicity [2]. Co-feeding soy meal exacerbates the urea toxicity because soyabeans contain urease, which exacerbates the toxicity by promoting the production of ammonia in addition to microbial urease [4]. After consumption, the urease enzyme in the rumen breaks down the urea, producing ammonia as a byproduct. The rumen bacteria then combines the ammonia with ketoacids generated from carbohydrates to synthesize proteins or amino acids.

When urea is consumed more quickly than it can be metabolized by rumen bacteria, poisoning results.

The extra ammonia generated in these situations enters the bloodstream and, at the cellular level, inhibits the Krebs cycle, impeding cellular respiration and ultimately resulting in anaerobic glycolysis, excessive lactic acid generation, and metabolic acidosis. Ammonia produces fake neurotransmitters at the neural level, which destabilizes neuronal conduction and manifests neurological abnormalities.In general, urea should not make up more than 3% of a ruminant's concentrate feed. In cattle, hazardous doses range from 0.3–0.5g/kg/day (or 120–200 g for a 400 kg cow) to 1-1.5g/kg/day (or 400–600 g for a 400 kg cow), which may be lethal. While sheep can consume 6% of their entire ration as urea as long as it is well blended with roughage and administered in sections throughout the day, horses seem to be tolerant of relatively large doses of urea [2].

Clinical signs

Toxicological symptoms could show up in a matter of minutes or hours. Blood ammonia levels, not rumen ammonia levels, determine when symptoms start and how severe they get. The animal may exhibit bruxism of the teeth, twitches of the face muscles, bloating, a stop to ruminating, increased salivation that appears frothy, abdominal pain that manifests as the animal kicking and struggling, increased bellowing, increased respiratory rate but labored breathing, coughing, and an increase in sensitivity to sound or movement. In less severe cases, the animal becomes lethargic, unconscious, and recumbent; in severe cases, the symptoms end with the animal's death.

Necropsy findings

Upon visual inspection, the carcass appears to swell and decompose quickly; the conjunctival mucus membrane is brick red in color; the ruminal contents smell strongly of ammonia; the liver and kidney are swollen; the rumen is bloated; and, especially in sheep, the trachea and bronchi may contain regurgitated or inhaled rumen contents [5]. Degenerative alterations in the brain are discernible histologically [4]. Serum, whole blood, urine, reticulo-ruminal contents of the animal, and suspected feed are among the samples that will be gathered for a toxicological analysis. When it comes time for analysis, the obtained samples should be thawed and promptly frozen. Samples taken from animals that have been dead for more than a few hours in a hot and muggy environment, or after 12 hours in a temperate temperature, are largely useless for diagnosis. At the field level, the differential diagnosis of the condition is aided by clinical findings such as alkaline ruminal fluid (~pH>8) without live microflora and elevated serum ammonia levels, among other things. The diagnosis is frequently based on a history of urea ingestion and suspicion of pasture land contamination.

Treatment

The initial stage of treatment is removing the possible cause of the poisoning. Sedatives may be utilized when an animal exhibits violent behavior that makes examination and treatment difficult. If given within 90 minutes of urea consumption, rumen infusion of 5% acetic acid (vinegar) up to 0.5-2 liters in sheep and goats and 2-8 liters in cattle may prove advantageous [5]. The urease enzyme's activity can be decreased by giving cold water to the animal, which not only dilutes the contents of the rumen but also decreases the temperature of the rumen medium. However, in extreme circumstances, rumen contents transfusions are required.

Antihistamines, intravenous calcium borogluconate and magnesium solutions to ease tetanic attacks, and fluid treatment (NS solution) to dilute systemic toxins and manage dehydration are advised. Diuretics can be used to control pulmonary oedema, however fluid therapy should be administered cautiously in this situation [6]. To improve the ruminal environment, a bolus of probiotics, amino acids, and yeast extract can be given.

References

1. Finch HJS, Samuel AM, Lane GPF. Fertilisers and manures. In: Finch HJS, Samuel AM, Lane GPF, editors. Lockhart & Wiseman's Crop Husbandry Including Grassland (Ninth Edition) [Internet]. Ninth Edit. Woodhead Publishing; 2014. p. 63–91. (Woodhead Publishing Series in Food Science, Technology and Nutrition). Available from: https://www.sciencedirect.com/science/article/pii/B9781782423713500047
2. Radostits OM, Gay CC, Hinchcliff KW, Constable PD. Diseases associated with inorganic and farm chemicals. In: Radostits OM, Gay CC, Hinchcliff KW, Constable PD, editors. Veterinary Medicine: A Textbook of the Diseases of Cattle, Horses, Sheep, Pigs and Goats. 10th ed. London: Elsevier Saunders; 2007. p. 1842–3.
3. Gimelli A, Pupin RC, Guizelini CC, Gomes DC, Franco GL, Vedovatto M, et al. Urea poisoning in cattle: A brief review and diagnostic approach. Pesqui Veterinária Bras. 2023;43:article ID 43:e07228.
4. Thompson LJ. Nonprotein Nitrogen Poisoning in Animals [Internet]. MSD Veterinary Manual. 2022. Available from: https://www.msdvetmanual.com/toxicology/ nonprotein-nitrogen-poisoning/nonprotein-nitrogen-poisoning-in-animals
5. Sharma SK, Joshi M, Kumar K, Paramjeet. Acute Urea Poisoning in Buffaloes: Case Study. Res Rev J Vet Sci. 2017;3(1):3–5.
6. The Merck veterinary manual [Internet]. Whitehouse Station, NJ : Merck & amp; Co., Inc.; 2013. 2588–2592 p. Available from: https://www.msdvetmanual.com/toxicology/household-hazards/overview-of-household-hazards

IV Miscellaneous

37

Euthanasia

Kumari Chandrakala

Key Points

- Animal euthanasia is the act of humanely killing animals, most commonly with injectable drugs.
- Euthanasia techniques vary by species, age, and the health status of the individual animal.
- Death must be confirmed before disposal of any animal remains.
- Animal remains must be disposed of in a legal manner that does not contaminate food sources or the environment.

Introduction

Euthanasia is the act of inducing humane death in an animal by a method that induces rapid loss of consciousness and death with a minimum of pain, discomfort, or distress. Euthanizing agents cause death by three basic mechanisms: (1) direct depression of neurons necessary for life function, (2) hypoxia, and (3) physical disruption of brain activity. Because loss of consciousness resulting from these mechanisms can occur at different rates, the suitability of a particular agent or method will depend on whether an animal experiences distress before loss of consciousness. Unconsciousness, defined as a loss of individual awareness, occurs when the brain's ability to integrate information is blocked or disrupted. Ideally, euthanasia techniques cause rapid loss of consciousness, followed by cardiac or respiratory arrest and death.

Protocol for dog euthanasia

The veterinarian should go into the room and, preferably, not leave again until the pet has passed (unless the owner requests time alone). Go in with the sedation and euthanasia solutions already in syringes in your pocket, or give them to your technician. Speak to the client and make a visual assessment of the pet.

Protocol for cattle euthanasia

Barbiturates and barbituric acid derivatives (acceptable), gunshot and penetrating captive bolts (acceptable with conditions). Penetrating and non-penetrating captive bolts are suitable for euthanasia of calves. Fast intravenous injections of a concentrated solution of magnesium sulphate or magnesium chloride or potassium chloride are also acceptable for the euthanasia of cattle.

Common Euthanasia Methods

1. Inhalation of anesthesia gas: acceptable with conditions for rodents and other small animals (< 7 kg). Typically used as part of a two-step process with a secondary physical method of euthanasia such as decapitation or cervical dislocation.
2. Inhalation of CO_2: acceptable with conditions, including the special considerations.
3. Immersion agents: e.g. MS 222/Tricaine. Acceptable for aquatic species, usually in connection with a secondary physical method.
4. Cervical Dislocation: acceptable for small birds, mice and immature rats. Requires training and should be performed under anesthesia unless specifically approved by the IACUC (The Intuitional Animal Care and Use Committee).
5. Decapitation: acceptable for rodents and small rabbits. Requires training; anesthesia recommended unless approved by the IACUC. Guillotines must be sharpened and adjusted frequently to ensure proper performance.
6. Injectable barbiturate agents: e.g. sodium pentobarbital, Euthasol®, Eutha 6®, Fatal Plus® - acceptable for most species.
7. Exsanguination/Cardiac Perfusion: acceptable with conditions; animals must be anesthetized.

Note: The IACUC strongly recommends the use of injectable anethestic agents (sodium pentobarbital, ketamine/xylazine, telazol, etc.) prior to cardiac perfusion.

Table. Agents and Methods of Euthanasia by Species

species	**Acceptable methods**[a]	**Acceptable conditions with conditions"b**
Aquatic invertebrates	S6.3c: Immersion in anesthetic solution (magnesium salts, clove oil, eugenol, ethanol)	S6.3: Adjunctive methods (second step) include 70% alcohol and neutral-buffered 10% formalin, pithing, freezing, boiling
Amphibians	S7.3: As appropriate by species-injected barbiturates, dissociative agents, and anesthetics as specified, topical buffered tricainemethanesulfonate or benzocaine hydrochloride	S7.3: As appropriate by species—inhaled anesthetics as specified, CO2, penetrating captive bolt or firearm, manually applied blunt force trauma to the head, rapid freezing of small (< 4 g [0.1 oz]) individuals where immediate death occurs
Avian species (*see also Poultry*, below)	S5: IV barbiturates	S5: Inhaled anesthetics, CO2, CO, N2, Ar, cervical dislocation (small birds and poultry), decapitation (small birds) S7.5: Gunshot (free-ranging birds)
Cats	S1: IV barbiturates, injected anesthetic overdose, Tributame, T61	S1: Barbiturates (alternative routes of administration), inhaled anesthetic overdose, COc, CO2c, gunshotc
Cattle	S3.2: IV barbiturates	S3.2: Gunshot, penetrating captive bolt
Dogs	S1: IV barbiturates, injected anesthetic overdose, Tributame, T61	S1: Barbiturates (alternative routes of administration), inhaled anesthetic overdose, COc, CO2c, gunshotc
Fish	S6.2: Immersion in buffered benzocaine or benzocaine hydrochloride, isoflurane, sevoflurane,quinaldine sulfate, buffered tricainemethanesulfonate, 2-phenoxyethanol, injected pentobarbital, rapid chilling (appropriate species), ethanol	S6.2: Eugenol, isoeugenol, clove oil, CO2-saturated water (aquarium-fish facilities/fisheries), decapitation/cervical transection/manually applied blunt force trauma followed by pithing or exsanguination, maceration (research setting), captive bolt (large fish)
Equids	S4: IV barbiturates	S 4: Penetrating captive bolt, gunshot
Marine mammals	S7.5(captive): Injected barbiturates (captive) S7.7 (free-ranging): Injected barbiturates or anesthetic overdose	S7.5 (captive): Inhaled anesthetics (captive) S7.7 (free-ranging): Gunshot, manually applied blunt force trauma, implosive decerebration
Nonhuman primates	S2.3, S7.4: Injected barbiturates or anesthetic overdose	S2.3, S7.4 (as appropriate by species): Inhaled anesthetic, CO, CO2

Poultry	S3.4: Injected barbiturates and anesthetic overdose	S3.4: CO2, CO, N2, Ar, low-atmospheric-pressure stunning, cervical dislocation (as anatomically appropriate), decapitation, manual blunt force trauma, electrocution, gunshot, captive bolt
Rabbits	S2.4: IV barbiturates	S2.4: Inhaled anesthetic overdose, CO2, cervical dislocation (as anatomically appropriate), penetrating captive bolt, nonpenetrating captive bolt
Reptiles	S7.3: As appropriate by species—injected barbiturates/buffered tricainemethanesulfonate, dissociative agents with adjunctive method and anesthetics as specified	S7.3: As appropriate by species—inhaled anesthetics as specified, CO2, penetrating captive bolt or firearm, manually applied blunt force trauma to the head, rapid freezing for animals < 4 g where immediate death occurs, spinal cord severance/destruction of brain (crocodilians)
Rodents	S2.2: Injected barbiturates and barbiturate combinations, dissociative agent combinations	S2.2: Inhaled anesthetics, CO2, CO, tribromoethanol, ethanol, cervical dislocation, decapitation, focused beam microwave irradiation
Small ruminants	S3.2: Injected barbiturates	S3.2: CO2 (goat kids), gunshot, penetrating captive bolt, nonpenetrating captive bolt (goat kids)
Swine	S3.3: Injected barbiturates	S3.3: CO2, CO, N2, Ar, gunshot, electrocution, penetrating captive bold, nonpenetrating captive bolt (piglets), manually applied blunt force trauma

Note: Initial "S" references with associated numbers in table entries refer to specific areas of more detailed information in the AVMA guidelines, available at www.avma.org/sites/default/files/2020-02/Guidelines-on-Euthanasia-2020.pdf

[a]Acceptable methods are those that consistently produce a humane death when used as the sole means of euthanasia.

[b]Acceptable methods with conditions are those that may require certain conditions to be met to consistently produce humane death, may have a greater potential for operator error or safety hazards, are not well documented in the scientific literature, or may require a secondary method to ensure death.

[c]Not recommended for routine use.

Death must be confirmed before disposal of any animal remains. A combination of criteria is most reliable in confirming death, including: Lack of pulse, breathing, corneal reflexes and response to firm toe pinch, inability to hear respiratory sounds and heartbeat by use of a stethoscope, graying of the mucous membranes, rigor mortis.

None of these signs alone, except rigor mortis, confirms death. Confirming death may best be accomplished by an adjunctive method (eg, thoracotomy, decapitation) performed after the loss of consciousness. Using an adjunctive method may be especially important when euthanizing ectothermic animals, because their heartbeat and respiration are difficult to assess. Animal remains must be disposed of in a legal manner that does not contaminate food sources or the environment.

References

1. AVMA Guidelines for the Euthanasia of Animals: 2013 Edition.
2. Guide for the care and use of Laboratory Animals, 8th Edition, 123-124.
3. Cia L. Johnson, DVM, Animal Welfare Division, American Veterinary Medical Association; Emily G. Patterson-Kane, PhD, ASPCReviewed/Revised Feb 2020 | Modified Nov 2022A,Reviewed/Revised Feb 2020 | Modified Nov 2022
4. www.avma.org/sites/default/files/2020-02/Guidelines-on-Euthanasia-2020.pdf.

Index